THE DOCTORS BOOK
OF
Home Remedies®
FOR
AIRBORNE ALLERGIES

Titles in
The Doctors Book of Home Remedies
series

Colds and Flu
Stronger Bones
Airborne Allergies
Sharper Memory

THE DOCTORS BOOK
OF
Home Remedies®
FOR
AIRBORNE ALLERGIES

100 new cures
for symptoms from pollen,
pets, dust, and mold

By the Editors of *PREVENTION*.
Edited by Mary S. Kittel

RODALE

Prevention and *The Doctors Book of Home Remedies* are registered trademarks of Rodale Inc.

Printed in the United States of America on acid-free ∞ , recycled paper ♻

Cover Designers: Lynn N. Gano and Tara Long

Library of Congress Cataloging-in-Publication Data

    The doctors book of home remedies for airborne allergies :
100 new cures for symptoms from pollen, pets, dust, and mold /
by the editors of Prevention ; edited by Mary S. Kittel.
       p.   cm.
  Includes index.
  ISBN 1–57954–211–5 paperback
  1. Hay fever—Popular works.   I. Kittel, Mary S.
II. Prevention Health Books.
RC590 .D63 2000
616.2'02—dc21   00–025360

Distributed to the book trade by St. Martin's Press

2 4 6 8 10 9 7 5 3 1   paperback

Visit us on the Web at www.rodaleremedies.com,
or call us toll-free at (800) 848-4735.

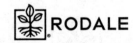

**WE INSPIRE AND ENABLE PEOPLE TO IMPROVE
THEIR LIVES AND THE WORLD AROUND THEM**

About *Prevention* Health Books

The editors of *Prevention* Health Books are dedicated to providing you with authoritative, trustworthy, and innovative advice for a healthy, active lifestyle. In all of our books, our goal is to keep you thoroughly informed about the latest breakthroughs in natural healing, medical research, alternative health, herbs, nutrition, fitness, and weight loss. We cut through the confusion of today's conflicting health reports to deliver clear, concise, and definitive health information that you can trust. And we explain in practical terms what each new breakthrough means to you, so you can take immediate, practical steps to improve your health and well-being.

Every recommendation in *Prevention* Health Books is based upon interviews with highly qualified health authorities, including medical doctors and practitioners of alternative medicine. In addition, we consult with the *Prevention* Health Books Board of Advisors to ensure that all of the health information is safe, practical, and up-to-date. *Prevention* Health Books are thoroughly factchecked for accuracy, and we make every effort to verify recommendations, dosages, and cautions.

The advice in this book will help keep you well-informed about your personal choices in health care—to help you lead a happier, healthier, and longer life.

Notice

This book is intended as a reference volume only, not as a medical manual. The information given here is designed to help you make informed decisions about your health. It is not intended as a substitute for any treatment that may have been prescribed by your doctor. If you suspect that you have a medical problem, we urge you to seek competent medical help.

Acknowledgments

The following writers and editorial researcher contributed to this book.

Writers: Brian Good; Paula Hunt; Kara Marantha Messinger; Colleen Pierre, R.D.; Betsy Torg
Editorial Researcher: Jennifer L. Kaas

We would like to thank the following health care professionals:
Sanford Archer, M.D.; Garrison Ayars, M.D.; Tammy Baker, R.D.; Betzy Bancroft; Kenneth Bock, M.D.; Mary Bove, N.D.; John Bower; Robert W. Boxer, M.D.; K. Shane Broughton, Ph.D.; Andrew Brown, M.D.; Doug Brugge, Ph.D.; Robert Bush, M.D.; Don Campbell; Peter J. Casano, M.D.; Alexander C. Chester, M.D.; Effie Poy Yew Chow, R.N., Dipl.Ac., Ph.D.; Valerie Cooksley, R.N.; William G. Crook, M.D.; Raymond Dattwyler, M.D.; Carrie Demers, M.D.; Merri Lou Dobler, R.D.; Victoria Edwards; Berrilyn J. Ferguson, M.D.; Trisha Lamb Feuerstein; Tiffany Field, Ph.D.; Linda B. Ford, M.D.; Kendall Gerdes, M.D.; Ralph T. Golan, M.D.; Barbara Gollman, R.D.; Gary N. Gross, M.D.; Elson Haas, M.D.; Wayne Hackett; Daniel Hamilos, M.D.; William Hostoffer, D.O.; Charles Jaffe, M.D., Ph.D.; Kathi Keville; Vasant Lad, M.A.Sc., B.A.M.S.; Charis Lindrooth, D.C.; Richard F. Lockey, M.D.; Richard Mabry, M.D.; Allan Magaziner, D.O.; Diana Marquardt, M.D.; Patricia McNally, M.D.; Chris Meletis, N.D.; Lisa Meserole, N.D.; Mary Ann Michelis, M.D.; William Mundy, M.D.; David C. Nieman, D.Sc.; Dean Ornish, M.D.; Terry Phillips, D.Sc., Ph.D.; Sandra Pinkham, M.D.; Robert Plancey, M.D.; Linda Rado, R.Y.T.; Phoebe Reeve; Judyth Reichenberg-Ullman, N.D.; Anthony R. Rooklin, M.D.; J. Loren Rosenberg, M.D.; Glenn S. Rothfeld, M.D.; John Steele; William W. Storms, M.D.; Steve L. Taylor, Ph.D.; Agatha Thrash, M.D.; Wellington S. Tichenor, M.D.; Michael Traub, N.D.; Normand Tremblay, M.D.; Andrew Weil, M.D.; John Weiler, M.D.; Gary Weinstock, M.D.; Betty Wray, M.D.; Stuart H. Young, M.D.; Janet Zand, O.M.D., L.Ac.; Irwin Ziment, M.D.

Contents

GETTING NATURAL RELIEF

While decongestants can make you irritated and antihistamines can make you drowsy, natural remedies can provide gentle, not to mention quick, resolutions to your symptoms with no side effects. Herbal experts, yoga teachers, holistic doctors, aromatherapists, and more offer you their favorite remedies to stop, or prevent, an allergy attack.

LIFESTYLE MATTERS

What you do day-to-day can help you avoid or lessen your allergies. These tips show how to build up your resistance through exercise, good sleeping habits, and proper care of your sinuses. Also learn how taking care of your emotions through relaxation and how developing positive attitudes can help you resist allergens.

ALTERNATIVE OPTIONS

Holistic healers may have a different approach than you've ever tried—one that can finally keep your sniffles and sneezes away. Consider seeing an expert in naturopathic medicine, homeopathy, aromatherapy, qigong, or herbalism. You'll learn more about alternative medicine practitioners and where to find them.

INDEX

Taking Control

Clearing Up the Facts

Historically, airborne allergy symptoms were called pollinosis. Then the terms *rose fever* and *hay fever* emerged, beginning the long chain of misnomers associated with airborne allergies.

The current medical term is *allergic rhinitis,* meaning an inflammation of the membrane lining the nose caused by substances light enough to be suspended in the air. Your body reacts to those airborne substances as if they were foreign invaders, and that's when inflammation occurs.

Although the habit of referring to allergic rhinitis by the catch-all term *hay fever* has stuck, it is as technically incorrect as the archaic terms *rose fever* and *pollinosis.* For starters, neither hay nor roses cause allergic reactions. And when a reaction occurs, fever is not one of the symptoms.

What you *can* expect from an allergic rhinitis attack is a nose running faster than you can say "pass the tissues," watery eyes, violent fits of sneezing, mucus buildup, and itching from the inner ear to the back of the throat.

It's probably good that the term *pollinosis* died out. Although pollen from grasses, trees, or weeds is a major allergy trigger, pollen is only the first part of the picture. Allergists consider reactions to such plants seasonal allergies since symptoms only develop when the allergen is in bloom. The second part of the picture is any agitator that you are exposed to in your environment all the time—found in things such as dust, mold, or pets. Doctors call reactions to these sources perennial allergens. About one-third of the allergy population suffers from seasonal allergies and one-third from perennial allergies. The remaining third—poor devils—suffer from both.

So why does your head turn into a bleary compression tank anytime between St. Patrick's Day and the first frost or anytime you encounter a four-footed friend? The mechanism behind allergic rhinitis is an odd one.

Case of Mistaken Identity

For reasons not fully understood, something that is usually harmless in the air—like dust mites, mold, pet dander, or pollen—is perceived to be dangerous by your immune system. Treating these substances like a friend-turned-foe, your T cells and B cells—usually reserved to fight dangerous pathogens—trigger a protein called immunoglobin E, or IgE.

Although your body doesn't respond with an allergic reaction the first time, it is now primed to do so at the next close encounter with the offending substance. Upon a second encounter, the IgE coats what are known as mast cells, and the interaction between IgE and the allergen leads to the release of chemicals from the mast cells. One particularly infamous chemical is histamine, which is largely responsible for the itching, burning, dripping, and sneezing that you experience. Worse yet, your mast cells continue to produce new chemicals—even when you are no longer in contact with the allergen—that perpetuate or worsen your symptoms.

Experts say that the number of Americans who experience this immune system quirk are well over 14 million. As if this party weren't big enough, the number of people with allergic rhinitis is currently on the rise.

The Plot Thickens

"Genetics help to predispose a person to allergies," says Charles Jaffe, M.D., Ph.D., an allergist and immunologist at the Allergy and Immunology Medical Group in San Diego. But genetics doesn't fully explain why allergic rhinitis is increasing among every socioeconomic status, age, and ethnic group in this country.

As ironic as it may be, it seems that modern medicine and modern technology might be the key to the rising incidence of allergic rhinitis.

One theory holds that we're more susceptible to allergens because we fight fewer diseases in childhood than we used to. "With vaccinations and early treatment of infectious diseases, it appears that we don't have the immune system revved up in the same way that it used to be," says Berrylin J. Ferguson, M.D., chief of the division of sino-nasal disorders, department of otolaryngology, at the University of Pittsburgh Medical Center in Pennsylvania.

Dr. Ferguson explains that since the TH1 cells that fight infection are not as active, the immune system activates TH2 cells—the ones that are overactive in allergic reactions.

Anthony R. Rooklin, M.D., clinical associate professor at the Thomas Jefferson University Hospital in Philadelphia and codirector of the division of allergy and clinical immunology at Crozer Chester Medical Center in Upland, Pennsylvania, puts it this way: "The unchallenged immune system is busy looking for something to do." This theory makes sense considering that allergic rhinitis is uncommon in more primitive cultures, which have a host of parasites and childhood diseases to contend with, keeping the immune system working on real illnesses rather than inventing them like it seems to do in the case of allergies.

Researchers have been able to detect variations of resistance within families, too. Studies performed in Italy found that the oldest child in a family is more likely to have allergies than a third, fourth, or fifth sibling. Since younger kids in larger families are exposed to more infections from their siblings, researchers suspect that their immune systems are stronger.

Sterile, tightly insulated homes may also be contributing to the rising incidence of allergies. In fact, 65 to 95 percent of children and young adults with asthma are allergic to multiple sources in their indoor environments. Dust mites thrive in wall-to-wall carpeting. Superinsulated houses seal in the molds, pollens, and pet dander. Furthermore, there are countless chemical irritants in cleaning products, self-care products, and paints and stains. Many of these chemicals can exasperate or trigger allergic symptoms.

Another theory about why allergies may be on the rise is related to ecology. "We have more exposure to hydrocarbons and petrochemicals now than we did in the past," says Dr. Rooklin. These airborne particulates, especially when combined with other allergens like pollen, stimulate the immune system to produce an allergic response.

Pollution could help explain why allergy is more common in urban areas than in rural, says Gary N. Gross, M.D., clinical professor of medicine at the University of Texas Southwestern Medical School in Dallas and executive vice president of the Joint Council of Allergy and Immunology.

Another concern is that planetary weather changes may be causing longer pollen seasons, says William Hostoffer, D.O., clinical assistant professor at Case Western Reserve University in Cleveland. This unnatural balance could be overwhelming the immune system.

You Are Still in Control

Genetic predisposition, immune system malfunction, planetary changes—these uncontrollable issues may seem overwhelming at first. But there is much that you can control. In fact, experts claim that with minimal effort, you can relieve, prevent, and possibly even cure allergic rhinitis. Consider the power you have over the following things.

• **Your attitude.** Ignoring your allergies is the worst approach you can take. First of all, there is no need to be miserable when there are countless simple, inexpensive ways to control your discomfort, as this book will show. Second, if ignored, your allergies will most likely get worse—thus becoming more difficult to reverse. Ignoring symptoms means not only more discomfort but also that allergies can sometimes predispose you to chronic conditions such as asthma, recurrent sinus infections, and secondary infections of the ear and throat. Once you acknowledge your allergies, you can develop a strategy to overcome them.

• **Identification and avoidance.** You may choose to see an allergist or a physician for testing. Seeing a doctor is recommended if you are unable to identify and control your allergies using self-care and if your allergies start to seriously interfere with your life. So before you start missing days of work, get to the bottom of your problem.

One of the first steps in managing your allergies is to figure out what sets them off. Trace Your Triggers on page 7 gives you tips and advice on how to determine if your allergens are caused by mold, pollen, dust, pets, chemicals, or foods. You will also learn if you are mistaking cold symptoms or sensitivity to a certain scent as an allergy attack.

• **Your living space.** The mainstay of self-care for allergies is what doctors refer to as environmental control. Basically, that's making changes in the surroundings where you spend most of your time—both at home and at work—to reduce your exposure to the allergens that offend your immune system.

"Environmental control is fairly simple, and you benefit by dramatically reducing the need for—or eliminating—medication," says Dr. Rooklin. So before rushing off to the drugstore for some over-the-counter allergy pills or to an allergist for allergy shots, consider the advice in Clear the Air on page 27. Learn how to live with a sneeze-producing pet, how to select the best air purifier, and how to take control of mold and dust.

• **Your diet.** If you've never thought of food as a weapon against allergies, think again. The Milk Makes Mucus, Fish

Fights Inflammation chapter on page 53 describes how hot peppers and horseradish work as expectorants to help you release mucus and how onions and pesto can stop a runny nose. Similarly, we'll show you how avoiding certain foods, like barbecued steaks and cheese, can help you avoid symptoms.

• **Prevention.** Experts will reveal how to strengthen your overall immunity through vitamins in Milk Makes Mucus, Fish Fights Inflammation on page 53; through herbs, delightful relaxation methods, and laughter in Getting Natural Relief on page 79; and through a daily routine that includes exercise and breathing techniques in Lifestyle Matters on page 103.

• **Self-care remedies.** Getting Natural Relief on page 79 not only offers suggestions for preventing symptoms but also tons of gentle techniques to stop discomfort on the spot, with no annoying side effects. Just a few of the breakthrough remedies you will be able to choose from include drinking herbal teas, soaking your feet in warm water, or engaging in a creative visualization technique that has shown an 85 percent success rate in actually curing allergies for good.

• **Your overall physical, mental, and emotional health.** In Lifestyle Matters on page 103, you'll be reminded that sometimes the simplest modifications in your daily routine can make a difference. For example, find out how sunglasses and shampoo can be two simple weapons in your fight against pollen and how the position in which you sleep can prevent congestion. Then, learn how to take steps to avoid smoking, worrying, and other unhealthy habits.

• **Seeking help.** Alternative health practitioners are savvy at helping you overcome your symptoms and at keeping them away without the use of drugs. Alternative Options on page 121 gives you the lowdown on what extra support you can get by visiting an Oriental medicine practitioner, an Indian doctor, an herbalist, a naturopath, and an aromatherapist.

Trace Your Triggers

"Diagnosing and treating allergies is essentially just a matter of careful observation and then avoidance."

—Diana Marquardt, M.D.,
chief of the allergy-immunology department at the University of California, San Diego, Medical Center

ACT ON YOUR ALLERGIES

Don't just learn to live with a runny nose and watery eyes. The effort you make to investigate and treat your symptoms will prevent future woes.

Finding the source of an allergy can take a lot of tedious trial and error. But in the long run, putting an end to chronic annoyances will do more than just make your life more pleasant.

"One of two things can happen with allergies. Either you can develop some form of resistance, or the allergy can continue to get more and more severe, and last for longer and longer periods of time," says Betty Wray, M.D. "In the case where symptoms become more severe, it becomes more difficult to reverse them."

"The most important reason to take allergies seriously is medical," says Dr. Wray. People with allergies suffer more than people without allergies when they catch colds and flu—they are more prone to sinus and ear infections. This happens because the respiratory tissues are already inflamed by the allergy.

Allergies can also escalate into serious medical conditions. For example, that "occasional" runny nose can turn into a chronic runny nose and a frequent headache and sinusitis. Ear infections accompanying sinus problems can lead to a ruptured ear canal. An even greater concern is that respiratory allergies can lead to asthma or worsen it.

Since determining the cause of your symptoms is the first step in resolving them, all of these potential complications add up to a really good reason to do some sleuthing.

Perhaps the best motivation of all is relief. After you've taken the time to figure out what you're up against, and you've taken steps to treat or avoid it, those symptoms can begin to disappear within days, says Dr. Wray.

> **—Betty Wray, M.D.,** *is the chief of allergy-immunology at the Medical College of Georgia in Augusta.*

DON'T TREAT YOUR ALLERGY LIKE A COLD

You have a runny nose and a sore throat. Is it just a cold, or have you developed an allergy?

Many people confuse the symptoms connected with colds with those connected with allergies. That confusion causes people to buy the wrong medications and, ultimately, delays the time it takes them to recover from whatever is ailing them.

According to Garrison Ayars, M.D., here are a few ways to identify your problem. "Itching is the one thing that almost always separates allergies from colds. If you have itchy eyes; an itchy throat; or dry, scratchy skin accompanying sniffles or a headache, you're likely to have an allergy. If you have a sore throat, stuffy nose, headache with a fever, or just feel weak in general, you're likely to have a cold."

Dr. Ayars says that colds should go away on their own within 7 to 10 days, while symptoms from allergies can persist for weeks or even months.

If you notice symptoms that are seasonal or that come

back at the same time year after year, he adds, that's another clue that what you're experiencing is caused by an allergy rather than by the common cold. Start by trying to identify the allergens rather than by wasting your money on cold medicine.

—Garrison Ayars, M.D., *is a clinical professor of medicine at the University of Washington School of Medicine in Seattle.*

START A SYMPTOM JOURNAL

Jotting down the who, what, where, when, and why of each allergy attack may be all you need to finally break the cycle.

If you're unsure of what's causing your allergy symptoms, get a notebook and start keeping track of everything around you and of everything that you are in contact with before each allergy attack.

"The secret to getting rid of your allergies," according to Diana Marquardt, M.D., "is really just a matter of good record keeping."

"No detail is too small," she says. Write down where you were, what plants or animals you may have been in contact with, what foods you ate, and what you were doing before the attack. Don't start out looking for oddball allergy sources. Most allergy symptoms are caused by four basic allergens: dust mites, mold, pollen, and pets.

If you can't come to any conclusion, continue to add more and more details to your journal. Eventually, says Dr. Marquardt, you'll begin to notice a pattern of some type—a time of day, a season of the year, a location at home or at work, or even a certain habit that might be responsible for your allergies.

"Once you've gotten down to what you might be allergic to," she says, "you have the power to eliminate the allergen from your environment."

—Diana Marquardt, M.D., *is the chief of the allergy-immunology department at the University of California, San Diego, Medical Center.*

DON'T LET FLOWER POWDER OVERPOWER

If it feels as if you're allergic to the entire great outdoors, chances are it's pollen.

Pollen is the most common adult allergen. If your allergic symptoms show up when you're outside, pollen should be your first suspect. The other possibility is mold, which gives you symptoms when you're exposed to specific organic material, like when you are gardening or camping next to a pond, rather than when you're just out walking or spending time outdoors.

If you believe a pollen is to blame, the plant source is probably one of three likely suspects: trees in early spring, grasses in midsummer, and weeds from late summer into fall.

"Since you can't exactly eliminate pollens from your environment, the best thing you can do is monitor pollen counts in the newspaper, and then on pollen-heavy days, spend the majority of your time indoors in air-conditioned or air-filtered buildings," says Allan Magaziner, D.O., who also recommends limiting the amount of time you spend outdoors early in the morning, when pollen counts are highest. Clear the Air on page 27 gives more specific tips on avoidance.

> —**Allan Magaziner, D.O.,** is the president and founder of the Magaziner Center for Wellness and Anti-Aging Medicine in Cherry Hill, New Jersey.

HOLD ON TO YOUR GREEN THUMB

Allergic to pollen? Don't give up flower gardening!

If you have allergies, that doesn't mean it's time to till under your petunias. "Most ornamental flowering plants don't release pollen into the air," says John Weiler, M.D. And even if they did, the pollen would be too heavy to be inhaled—unless you stick your nose directly into the plant.

"Instead of the airborne method, the decorative flowers that people keep in their yards rely on insects for pollination. The plants that release pollen into the air are generally not ornamental; they're less desirable plants like ragweed instead of more attractive flowering plants like roses or daisies."

According to Dr. Weiler, the most common sources of airborne pollens typically include trees, grasses, and weeds rather than your prizewinning chrysanthemums.

> —**John Weiler, M.D.,** is a professor of allergy at the University of Iowa in Iowa City.

DON'T ASSOCIATE WITH STRANGE FUNGI

Basements, bathrooms, and other moist, dark, nooks in your house are usually the suspected places when it comes to mold. But your mold allergy is more likely to be triggered outside of your home.

Fuzzy black stuff is in countless more places than just in the back of the refrigerator. So keeping a spick-and-span house won't solve the problem if you're allergic to mold. That's because it grows where your broom can't go—on trees, on crops, and in soil where it's needed by nature to break down organic material.

Mold is a necessary component of life on this planet—something that makes some people with allergies want to relocate to someplace like Jupiter. "It's not even killed by frost," says Peter J. Casano, M.D., "so mold spores lurk outside almost year-round—except when snow is on the ground."

Weather is the best determinant of whether or not mold is your foe. "If your allergy symptoms last most of the year, but tend to flare up when it rains a lot—like in early spring when pollen isn't a big problem yet—then it's likely you're allergic to mold," says Dr. Casano.

Although trying to eliminate mold spores from your environment is impossible, you can avoid the places where they reproduce. Dr. Casano recommends wearing a face mask whenever you're raking leaves or grass, mowing the lawn, or doing anything else that disturbs the soil and releases mold spores into the environment. That goes for gardeners whenever they are planting crops or mixing the compost pile.

You should also watch out for especially damp areas when hiking or camping. Dark areas with rotting logs or stagnant water can also be home to a number of different types of mold, so don't set up camp next to a pond, says Dr. Casano. See Clear the Air on page 27 for more tips on mold avoidance.

—Peter J. Casano, M.D., *is an allergy specialist and otolaryngologist in Jackson, Mississippi.*

NIGHT TIME IS MITE TIME

It's no wonder you sneeze and wheeze while you snooze. You can't see them, but there are thousands of tiny creatures keeping you company in bed.

Dust mites are microscopic organisms that live in our homes and eat the dead skin that falls from our bodies as we move around. While humans aren't allergic to the mites themselves, we are allergic to their waste and by-products.

"People whose allergies are more pronounced indoors, or who are especially congested when they sleep and wake up, are likely to be allergic to dust mites," says Diana Marquardt, M.D. "Allergic reactions are worse at night because that's when they're around the mites."

Give up on the idea that you can rid your home of dust mites—99 percent of homes contain them, even the most fanatically sanitary ones. But you can make the rooms you spend the majority of your time in, especially your bedroom, as spartan as possible, says Dr. Marquardt. "You should only have items in the room that you can pick up and wash in hot water—including upholstery, curtains, and rugs—and you should wash these materials every week, at best."

See Clear the Air on page 27 for tips on mite control.

—Diana Marquardt, M.D., *is the chief of the allergy-immunology department at the University of California, San Diego, Medical Center.*

WHEN YOU CAN'T NAP WITH A FRIEND

It shouldn't take much effort to figure out if you're allergic to cats or dogs—unless you've been around one or the other all your life.

There's been a cat or a little dog sleeping at the foot of your bed for as long as you can remember. Come to think of it, for as long as you've had that perennially stuffy nose. Why didn't you make the connection?

You may have had low-grade symptoms for a long time, but they were too subdued to make anything of them. "If you have constant daily exposure to pet dander, you do develop some allergic immunity on your own to the allergen," says Normand Tremblay, M.D. "That means you won't have immediate reactions to the allergen, but you could still have chronic low-grade symptoms that you may consider a normal part of day-to-day life."

You may also not have suspected your pet because your

allergy crept up very slowly over time. It can take up to 2 years of exposure before you actually have symptoms, which can include asthma, chronic sinus congestion, sinus infection, and a chronically stuffy nose.

Don't make the mistake of thinking that you won't have allergies because you choose a cat or a dog that is supposed to be a nonallergenic breed. Although the fur of some breeds carries less dander than that of others, your immune system can overreact to any animal's dander, saliva, and dried urine.

Dr. Tremblay says that whatever the case, you're going to have to wean your pet from the bedroom. Do it gradually, so you both can adjust.

For tips on eliminating pet allergens, see Clear the Air on page 27.

—Normand Tremblay, M.D., *is an allergist practicing in Fort Worth, Texas.*

CONSIDER YOUR EXOTIC PET

Most people suspect their pooches, but did you know that your other pets could be causing your allergies?

It's not just cats and dogs that release allergens like hair and dander into your home. Any animal with fur—including mice, hamsters, rabbits, horses, and monkeys—can be the cause of your stuffy nose.

And mammals aren't alone. The feathers from birds, dust from snake and reptile tanks, and algae from fish tanks could also be to blame, says Betty Wray, M.D.

Like allergies to cats and dogs, allergies to exotic animals include symptoms like a runny nose, itchy eyes, sneezing, and labored breathing.

If getting rid of your pet isn't an option, Dr. Wray says, it's best to keep the animal out of the rooms where you spend the most time and to thoroughly clean up after it, wearing gloves and a mask if necessary.

It's also important to prevent algae from growing in your fish tank by keeping the tank away from direct sunlight, changing filters when needed, and even buying fish that eat algae. You should also clean the insides of cages for small animals and birds frequently, and replace the animal's bedding as often as possible—something that will also help to cut down on the number of allergens released into your home.

—Betty Wray, M.D., *is the chief of allergy-immunology at the Medical College of Georgia in Augusta.*

FOOD ALLERGIES ARE NOTHING TO SNEEZE AT

That runny nose and congestion that you suspect as an airborne allergy may actually be an allergic reaction to food.

Usually, the symptoms associated with food allergies are headaches, rashes, diarrhea, and vomiting. But in some cases, respiratory problems like excess mucus in the nose and throat or labored breathing also result, according to William G. Crook, M.D.

Roughly 1 percent of all adults are allergic to some type of food, and many people have sensitivities to foods that also cause respiratory problems. It's possible that you could have a food allergy *and* hay fever. Many people who are allergic to one allergen are also allergic to other allergens, which can make their symptoms even worse.

If you haven't been able to nail your allergen to pollen, mold, dust mites, or pet dander, it's possible that your diet is the culprit.

"If you're allergic to a specific food like broccoli or rhubarb that you don't eat every day," says Dr. Crook, "you'll know about your allergy immediately, because symptoms will show up as soon as the food enters your mouth."

Finding more common allergens requires the effort of an at-home diet that seeks to determine which foods you're allergic to by a process of elimination. "First, look at the foods you eat most frequently," says Dr. Crook. "Things like dairy products, wheat, yeast, corn, eggs, fruit juices, and products with food colors and dyes. Then, pick a group of foods and completely eliminate it from your diet for at least a week."

If your allergic symptoms disappear, you've found the culprit. If they don't disappear, pick a different group of foods and repeat the process. Continue until you find the allergen.

Just be sure not to experiment with any foods you've had a severe allergic reaction to in the past. Dr. Crook warns that just a few bites of common allergens like peanuts, dairy products, or seafood can be fatal to certain individuals.

—William G. Crook, M.D., *is an allergy specialist in Jackson, Tennessee, and author of* Detecting Your Hidden Allergies.

ARE YOU IRRITATED?

They may not be actual allergens, but the irritants you're exposed to each day can leave you feeling just as miserable—and can actually trigger symptoms similar to allergic reactions.

Your eyes are burning. You can't breathe well. You're sneezing. Allergies? Maybe not.

"Things like chalk dust, pepper, chemicals, and petroleum products are all sources of irritation but are not actual allergens for most people," says J. Loren Rosenberg, M.D. "Allergic reactions occur when you are exposed to a substance that stimulates your immune system to produce allergic antibodies. With irritants, your nasal membrane is stimulated, but there's no actual immune system response going on within your body, even though your symptoms are similar."

Anything other than mold, dust mites, pollen, and animal dander that causes symptoms of allergies is most likely an irritant. The good news about irritants is that they are easy to manage since they often show up only in certain situations—for instance, chalk dust will most likely show up only near chalkboards and pepper only in the kitchen. And their symptoms only last a brief time compared to allergy symptoms, which can last hours or days.

You can learn to stand downwind when you're filling up your car if the smell of gas is an irritant, or you can try to avoid using dry erase markers. Trying to avoid airborne pollens is much more difficult.

"As long as you put your mind to it, avoidance is easy when you have something very specific within your living space that you know you're allergic to," says Dr. Rosenberg.

—J. Loren Rosenberg, M.D., *is an allergy specialist and assistant clinical professor of medicine at the University of Medicine and Dentistry of New Jersey Robert Wood Johnson Medical School in New Brunswick.*

ARE YOU ALLERGIC TO YOUR JOB?

You feel fine at home but lately, work seems to be getting the best of you. Your workplace could be the source of your headaches and congestion.

Workplace allergens are fairly common. The bad news is that if you're exposed to a large number of allergens at work, your allergies can get worse over time or from over-exposure, causing you to develop allergies to things that never used to bother you.

This is especially true if you're working someplace where you're surrounded by mold, dust, pollen, animal dander, or chemicals (such as an auto body shop, a beauty shop, a construction site, or a farm) on a daily basis. But it can even happen in business settings, where you might be exposed to stale, moldy air and not even know it.

If you already know what you're exposed to at work, the best step is simply to get rid of those allergen-producing elements, Doug Brugge, Ph.D., says. If that's not possible, look at the different types of ventilation available, and choose one that may help to clear the contaminants from the air.

"If avoidance and ventilation aren't possible, your last step should be personal protective equipment," adds Dr. Brugge. "Try wearing a face mask, gloves, and long sleeves to cut down on exposure, and change your clothes and take a shower once you get home." You can even wear protective eyewear and a hat or a hood if necessary.

Since face masks and goggles are not practical in an office, white-collar workers must depend on their detective skills, especially if they are not sure what they're allergic to. "Search for water damage in and around the building you work in. Then, walk through the halls looking for discolored areas, musty smells, or stains on the ceiling panels—all of which could indicate mold growth.

"Start with the areas you spend the most time in, and work backward from there," he says. If you don't come up with anything from there, have the building engineer examine the ventilation system, which can harbor colonies of mold spores. Then look at any recent renovation, freshly painted areas, and new or old carpets—all of which release allergens and irritants into your environment.

—Doug Brugge, Ph.D., *is an assistant professor in the department of family medicine and community health at Tufts University in Medford, Massachusetts.*

EDUCATE YOUR NOSE

Many people shun strong odors and substances that cause their noses to become stuffy or runny, fearing an allergy attack. But to set the record straight, runny noses may have nothing to do with allergies.

If your nose begins to run every time you go into an air-conditioned room, it may seem like you are allergic to something in the room. It may also seem like you are suffering from allergies if you get a runny nose when you go outside in the winter, drink alcohol, read certain types of newspaper, or come into contact with certain scents. What you are most likely suffering from instead of allergic rhinitis is a condition known as vasomotor rhinitis.

"Vasomotor rhinitis is an unusual sensitivity that some people have to noxious substances in the environment," says John Weiler, M.D. "It causes a runny nose and congestion, but it's not the result of an actual allergy to any substance." Aside from things like tobacco smoke and perfume, vasomotor rhinitis can also be brought on by high humidity levels, chemical fumes, and stress.

The difference between an actual allergy and vasomotor rhinitis is that an allergy involves an immune system response within the body, whereas vasomotor rhinitis is probably caused solely by an unusual nervous system activity. The problem, though, is that certain substances that cause allergies can also cause vasomotor rhinitis. Therefore, the secret to successfully treating your symptoms is figuring out which condition you really have.

According to Dr. Weiler, if your nose is running but you aren't experiencing any itchiness in your eyes, nose, ears, or throat, then you are probably suffering from vasomotor rhinitis rather than an allergy.

In that case, the only thing you can really do to solve the problem is to find out what substance is causing the reaction and then avoid it. Don't waste your money on decongestants or antihistamines.

—John Weiler, M.D., *is a professor of allergy at the University of Iowa in Iowa City.*

EXHAUSTED? ROLL UP YOUR WINDOW

Starting the workday with a breath of fresh air sounds healthy—unless the air blowing in your face is fresh off the interstate.

Commuting to work is more than just a drag. It's also a source of early-morning headaches and breathing problems for an increasing number of people.

Allan Magaziner, D.O., warns commuters who drive to work with their windows open that exhaust fumes from busy rush-hour streets could be the cause of many early-morning allergy symptoms.

People who live by interstates or who are exposed to large amounts of exhaust pollution suffer from many of the same allergic symptoms as people with dust mite or pollen allergies. The exhaust fumes can act either as an allergen or as an irritant, causing symptoms like congestion, itchy eyes, runny nose, and headaches.

To combat the problem, Dr. Magaziner recommends driving with your car windows up and (if it's not cold outside) with your air conditioner on.

He also advises that you drive on less congested streets, avoid rush-hour traffic, and even buy an air filter for your car.

That's especially important advice for anyone who feels ill for the first hour or so after getting to work and for the first hour or so after coming home in the evening, when symptoms from an exhaust fume allergy would be at their peak.

—Allan Magaziner, D.O., *is the president and founder of the Magaziner Center for Wellness and Anti-Aging Medicine in Cherry Hill, New Jersey.*

WASH AWAY CHEMICAL SENSITIVITIES

Concern for the environment isn't the only reason to switch to more natural household products. Switching floor cleaners may be all you need to do to stop wheezing when you're doing housework.

The average home is filled with thousands of different chemicals designed for everything from polishing silver to cleaning carpet stains. But these chemicals also have a more dubious role—that of potential allergen or irritant.

"Many people suffer from chemical irritations without even being aware of having an actual sensitivity," says Peter J. Casano, M.D.

Unexplained rashes, itchiness, headaches, sinus problems, congestion, and nausea can all be caused by even the most innocuous-looking bottle of solvent under your bathroom sink. The only way to know which cleaner may be leaving your sink looking good but you feeling bad is the elimination method.

"You can't stop cleaning, so the trick to finding potential allergens is to start with the simplest possible products and make observations," says Dr. Casano.

Gather all your cleaners together and move them out of your primary living space—which includes the area under the kitchen sink and bathroom sink. Then, switch to milder detergents and cleaners, looking for items that are free of perfumes and dyes, which can act as potential irritants and make your existing allergies even worse.

"If your symptoms disappear with the mild cleansers, you'll know you're allergic to some type of chemical," says Dr. Casano. To find out which one, slowly add back one cleaning product per week to your daily routine and monitor your symptoms to see if they reappear.

—Peter J. Casano, M.D., *is an allergy specialist and otolaryngologist in Jackson, Mississippi.*

Clear the Air

"The classic recommendation for hay fever is to reduce your exposure to pollen and your other triggers as much as possible. It may not be practical to actually move to another part of the country, but there are countless other ways to avoid allergens."

—Lisa Meserole, N.D.,
research consultant and faculty member at Bastyr University and a naturopathic physician at Healing Arts in Seattle

MAKE MAJOR CLEANING A SEASONAL HABIT

Remember spring cleaning? It's one of the best ways to keep allergens under control.

Superthorough cleaning is an effective way of decontaminating the home from allergens. People used to literally take everything out of a room, wash down the walls, wash the floors, and beat the carpet—leaving it outside to air out, which probably killed the mites.

Allergy researcher Richard F. Lockey, M.D., has noticed that we've strayed a long way from this kind of judicious housekeeping. "When you go into homes today, they're really not cleaned very well." But with both heads of the household working, this is understandable, he says. If you can find the time or if you can pay someone to "spring clean" at least once a year, however, you'll be doing your health a service.

"Studies have shown that rigorous cleaning and dust mite–control methods effectively decrease allergen exposure and improve health," says Dr. Lockey.

A rigorous cleaning includes washing all surfaces—cupboards, walls, window ledges, countertops, baseboards—with a chlorine bleach solution to remove animal, cockroach, and mold allergens. Furniture should be cleaned with a damp cloth, and carpets and upholstery should be vacuumed using a vacuum cleaner with a double bag or a HEPA filter, which picks up nearly 100 percent of airborne allergens. (HEPA stands for high-efficiency particulate air.)

—Richard F. Lockey, M.D., *is a professor of medicine, pediatrics, and public health at the University of South Florida College of Medicine in Tampa.*

MASK YOUR ALLERGENS

Wearing a respiratory mask isn't the height of fashion, but it can make you breathe easier.

You might consider wearing a respiratory mask to reduce the amount of allergens you inhale during the pollen season or even when you are dusting and vacuuming.

"Wearing a mask can make a big difference if you get the right kind," says Stuart H. Young, M.D. "Those little paper ones you get at the hardware store are better than nothing, but you should get something that is specifically for allergies."

Allergy masks come in a range of prices and styles, from inexpensive disposable models to more expensive models with replaceable HEPA (high-efficiency particulate air) filters. You can purchase masks through specialty allergy companies or in drugstores. Commercial masks with charcoal filters to eliminate fumes can be purchased at art supply stores.

Make sure that the mask fits snugly but comfortably around your nose and mouth, so that contaminated air doesn't enter. You can even wear your mask outdoors when gardening or doing yard work. Just don't forget to take it off before you run to the store for a new rake.

—Stuart H. Young, M.D., *is the director of Allergy Fellow's Clinical Education in the department of internal medicine at Mount Sinai Hospital in New York City and coauthor of* Allergies: The Complete Guide to Diagnosis, Treatment, and Daily Management.

MITE-PROOF YOUR SLEEPING SPACE

Dust mites are public enemy number one when it comes to indoor allergens, so make banishing them from your bedroom a priority.

Dust mites are tiny critters that feed on live human skin cells and other debris. You'll find them everywhere you are, especially in your bed. In fact, a double bed can accommodate nearly two million dust mites. You'll never get rid of all of them, but you can reduce their numbers significantly in a number of ways," says Linda B. Ford, M.D.

Dr. Ford recommends starting your dust mite offensive by encasing mattresses, box springs, and pillows in allergen-free impermeable covers to create a barrier between you and the mites, thus decreasing their food supply. These covers can be purchased in drugstores and department stores.

It is important to strip your bed linens once a week to strip away mite exposure. To kill the mites, you must wash the linens in water that is at least 130°F. Be sure to dry them thoroughly. If you have a pollen allergy, don't dry them outside.

Water beds can be a healthy alternative to a mattress and box springs since there is no padding or stuffing for the mites to live in. But you must still wash linens and mattress pads in 130°F water every week and dry them thoroughly. Also, be on the lookout for any leaks or water that collects near your water bed, since dust mites—and mold, too—love moisture.

Aggressive mite control also involves clearing away

clutter—especially items with fabric where dust can settle. Remove upholstered furniture and bric-a-brac from the bedroom.

Dust mites will even inhabit the stuffed animals on your bed. If you can't toss Teddy in the washer, Dr. Ford suggests putting him in the freezer for one hour every week—until "crisp." This will give mites a fatal chill.

> **—Linda B. Ford, M.D.,** *is a physician and chief*
> *executive officer at the Asthma and Allergy Center in*
> *Papillion, Nebraska, and past president of the*
> *American Lung Association.*

BAG THE CARPET

Replacing carpet with wood or vinyl
floor covering will get rid of a prolific
allergen producer.

Shag, sculptured, olive green, or floral. Your taste in carpeting doesn't matter to the mold, dust mites, and animal dander that find carpeting a great place to hang out.

"Carpeting and carpet pads are a major source of allergens," says Robert W. Boxer, M.D., "and they should be removed, especially from the bedroom, if you have allergies. They harbor mold, bacteria, dust mites, and everything else you track into your house on your shoes. Every time you walk on a carpet, you kick up whatever is in there."

Hardwood and vinyl floor coverings are good alternatives to carpet because they are not conducive to mold growth, and allergens can be easily removed with a damp mop. Even if you vacuum your carpet regularly, says Dr. Boxer, you can actually make the problem worse because unless you have a vacuum with a HEPA (high-efficiency particulate air) filter, you're pulling out the dust and putting it right back into the air. And even a HEPA-filtered vacuum cleaner isn't going to remove all allergen particles from the carpet—especially cat dander.

If you're a die-hard carpet fan, you can reduce allergens by using a cleaner containing benzyl benzoate. Be sure to follow the manufacturer's instructions.

In the end, you're better off going bare, says Dr. Boxer. If you want something fuzzy under your feet, get plush slippers.

—Robert W. Boxer, M.D., *is an allergist in Skokie, Illinois.*

KEEP ALLERGENS AWAY FROM THE WINDOW

Fabric drapes and venetian blinds not only keep the light out of your home but also keep the allergens in.

Drapes collect dust, dust mites, and other airborne allergens like cat dander and cockroach waste. According to Andrew Brown, M.D., it is especially important to remove drapes from a bedroom since that's where you spend most of your time.

If you're in the redecorating mood, consider replacing dry-clean-only drapes with drapes that can be washed once a week in hot water. Although venetian blinds don't contribute dust to the air as do fabric window coverings, they do become dusty. You can help control the amount of particles collected on blinds by vacuuming or washing them every week, too.

If you spot condensation on your windows, check to see

that mold isn't growing on the drapes. If so, the drapes should be dry-cleaned or washed in hot water immediately.

To help keep the mold problem from recurring, keep drapes open during the day so that condensed air doesn't form on the windows. Another alternative is to reseal your windows or to install energy-saving double windows to minimize the creation of moisture.

—**Andrew Brown, M.D.,** *is an allergist in Gadsden, Alabama.*

CONTROL THE ALLERGENS IN YOUR BASEMENT

To prevent your house from becoming a breeding ground for allergens, you need to start at the bottom.

Don't let your basement be a welcoming environment for mold, mildew, and dust mites.

A prime suspect is water in your basement. "Water can seep into walls and climb up into baseboards, bringing mold along with it," warns Daniel Hamilos, M.D.

"Carpeting laid directly on concrete floors in basements can be a real problem, too," he adds, "because moisture develops between the two surfaces." Damp carpeting is an ideal breeding ground for dust mites and mold, especially if your basement is warm or not well-ventilated.

Tear out old carpeting and install an insulated floor. If you don't have air-conditioning in your basement, run a dehumidifier to keep the relative humidity level below 50 percent.

If your clothes dryer is located in the basement, dust can also be a problem because it blows lint and fiber dust into the air. The dryer hose should be sealed tightly so that particles don't escape back into your house, and it should ventilate to the outside (preferably, not under a bedroom window).

—Daniel Hamilos, M.D., *is an associate professor of medicine at the Washington University School of Medicine and at the Barnes-Jewish Hospital, both in St. Louis, Missouri.*

CLOSE THE DOOR ON POLLEN

Try these strategies so that your home doesn't become as populated by pollen as the field behind your house.

If you keep your windows open, depending on the velocity and direction of the wind, the normally absent or low pollen count *inside* your house can soon equal the *outside* pollen count. "Keeping the windows and doors of your house closed is the best and simplest way to limit your exposure," says allergist Robert W. Boxer, M.D.

When you do need to air out the house, Dr. Boxer recommends that you open the windows for an hour or two in the afternoon (especially on a rainy day), when pollen counts are low. Ideally, do it when the person who is allergic is not at home, and run an air-filter system immediately after closing the windows.

Additionally, don't let pollen hitch a ride into your home on its inhabitants. When you or your family members have been out on a high-pollen day, leave your shoes and outer clothing in the garage or in a closet away from the bedroom. Also, take a shower and wash your hair before you go to bed so that you won't breathe pollen all night long.

Pollen will also cling to animal fur so don't play doorman to your pet during pollen season. Keep Fluffy and Fido either inside or outside.

—Robert W. Boxer, M.D., *is an allergist in Skokie, Illinois.*

KEEP YOUR COOL WITH AIR-CONDITIONING

Air-conditioning isn't just a luxury to help you withstand the heat of the summer. If you have allergies, it's a powerful defense.

For starters, running an air conditioner rather than opening the windows in hot months means that less outdoor pollen and mold are entering your home. Air conditioners also remove contaminants from the air, especially systems that have high-quality filters. But the ultimate function of air conditioners when it comes to controlling allergens is reducing humidity.

The key factor in controlling mold growth and dust mites is to keep the relative humidity below 50 percent. To adjust your air conditioner to the proper humidity, monitor levels with a hygrometer (which can be purchased for under $25 at a hardware store), says consultant John Bower.

But your air conditioner will do more harm than good if it's not well-maintained. Window units can become contaminated with mold because moisture condenses on the coils and filter or collects in the drip pan. Make sure that they are draining correctly and that the filter isn't clogged with debris. Dr. Bower also recommends that you run the unit in the recirculate mode continuously, if possible.

Central air-conditioning systems should be checked every year by a professional to ensure that the vents are moisture-free inside and that the filter is clean.

—**John Bower** *is the owner of the Healthy House Institute, a resource center for designers, architects, contractors, and homeowners in Bloomington, Indiana; and author of several books, including the* Healthy House *series.*

FLUSH OUT BATHROOM MOLD

Your favorite room for pampering yourself is also, unfortunately, a favorite hiding place for mold, so take extra care keeping the bathroom clean and dry.

Some mold is visible, like the mold you find on your shower curtain or in the grout. Other mold might be under the floor, especially by the bathtub and toilet if they aren't sealed properly.

Even if you can't see or smell mold, there's a good chance it's there, says Raymond Dattwyler, M.D. That's because the moisture and warmth in a bathroom are mold's favorite breeding conditions.

A good local ventilation system that draws moisture outside after a bath or shower is critical to reducing the humidity in your bathroom, and it prevents moisture from circulating throughout the rest of your house.

Upkeep makes a difference, too. Regrout or recaulk areas where water is leaking. Use a washable shower curtain or liner and toss it in the laundry every week. Piles of wet towels are a favorite mold habitat and contribute to the room's humidity, so hang them up to dry or remove them from the room.

To kill mold on the spot, Dr. Dattwyler recommends cleaning bathroom surfaces once a week with a solution of 1/4 cup of chlorine bleach diluted in 1 gallon of water. To prevent mold from developing, wipe down the shower stall and bathroom walls with a squeegee or a towel after each use to remove water and condensation.

—Raymond Dattwyler, M.D., *is a professor of medicine and head of the division of allergy and clinical immunology at the State University of New York at Stony Brook.*

MAINTAIN YOUR DUCTS

Don't let the saying "out of sight, out of mind" be the rule with your home's duct system. It can be a sneaky source of mold and pollen allergens.

We usually don't think about the system that conducts hot and cold air through our homes, since it's in the basement, hidden inside closets, or behind walls. But according to consultant John Bower, ductwork should be cleaned as needed and inspected once a year.

A properly functioning duct system is free of leaks and debris. A clean, efficient system will not only reduce the amount of allergens in your home but will also probably reduce your energy bill. To keep air leaks out of ducts, Bower recommends sealing them with water-based duct-sealing mastics rather than with duct tape, which can fall off in less than a year.

Standard furnaces are equipped with particulate filters that keep big particles out of the furnace's fan motor but don't do much for your allergies. Better heating systems (as well as air-conditioning systems) have at least electrostatic filters that charge and trap tiny particles like animal dander. But for superior allergy protection, install a HEPA (high-efficiency particulate air) or medium-efficiency filter.

Unfortunately, installing a HEPA filter may mean having to modify the ductwork and fan motor; adding a medium-efficiency filter, like an electrostatic variety, requires minimal modification.

—**John Bower** *is the owner of the Healthy House Institute, a resource center for designers, architects, contractors, and homeowners in Bloomington, Indiana; and author of several books, including the* Healthy House *series.*

SERVE UP CLEAN AIR

For a mold-controlled kitchen, keep the surroundings dry and rot-free.

Since water and warmth are conducive to mold growth, you need to take precautions in your kitchen. Start with the sink area. Resolve any leaks or condensation on the pipes. Wash your sponges and dishcloths in hot water once a week and dry them thoroughly since they are home to mold as well as bacteria.

Next, think about your waste material. Recycling may help the Earth, but it won't help your allergies if you store dirty food containers in the kitchen. Either wash them thoroughly or keep them outside.

"Don't let food rot in the kitchen garbage, either," says Raymond Dattwyler, M.D. "Take it outside if what's inside goes bad." Refrigerated food can release mold spores, too, so periodically check containers to make sure that there's nothing growing in them.

"Clean the seal around your refrigerator door and the drip pan on the bottom with ¼ cup of chlorine bleach diluted in 1 gallon of water," says Dr. Dattwyler. "You can also use this solution to wipe down countertops, inside cupboards, sinks, and other surfaces to prevent mold from growing."

—**Raymond Dattwyler, M.D.,** *is a professor of medicine and head of the division of allergy and clinical immunology at the State University of New York at Stony Brook.*

PUT A LEASH ON CAT AND DOG ALLERGENS

Control your four-footed companion's dander, and you might not have to give him up.

Many allergists will tell you plainly that if you're allergic to animals, you should find your pet another home. The next best bet is to keep it outside. But you might be able to keep it inside if you follow the basic rules.

"Keep pets out of the bedroom, and keep them clean," says Linda B. Ford, M.D.

You may be having a reaction to your pet's dander—skin cells he sheds on a regular basis—or you may be reacting to his saliva or urine. Giving your pet a bath once a week with a pet shampoo, a grooming solution, or even just plain water can help. Weekly bathing can remove up to 85 percent of his dander. Chances are kitty isn't thrilled about being immersed, so giving her a full body rub with a warm, wet washcloth is a good alternative.

Even washing your pet every week, however, will not get rid of all of the dander. "Animal dander is very light and airborne," says Dr. Ford, "so you'll need to have a good ventilation system, like central air or a portable air cleaner with a HEPA filter." (HEPA stand for high-efficiency particulate air.) Studies have shown these to be very effective in reducing the amount of cat and dog dander in homes, especially if the pet is not allowed in the room where the system is installed and if there is no carpet on the floor.

The allergens that pets give off remain active for months, and it can take even longer for your body to adjust. So even if you aggressively clean and give your pet a new home, don't expect your symptoms to cease right away.

—Linda B. Ford, M.D., *is a physician and chief executive officer at the Asthma and Allergy Center in Papillion, Nebraska, and past president of the American Lung Association.*

STAY A STEP AHEAD OF ROACHES

Cockroaches are more than creepy; they are potential allergens. Eliminating their food and water sources can prevent their dreaded visit to your home.

Allergens from cockroaches—found in their bodies, saliva, and feces—can be inhaled. Although cockroaches can be found throughout the house, focus your antibug campaign in the kitchen, where they are most likely to convene.

Eliminate their food supply by keeping kitchen counters, floors, and sinks free of food, food splatters, and crumbs. Confine your eating to one room of the house so that cockroaches are not snacking in front of the television or in your bedroom. Cut off their water supply by checking sinks and refrigerators for leaks and by getting rid of dirty rags and damp paper products, like newspapers and cardboard containers.

If a few bugs have already paid you a visit, sprinkle boric acid around infested areas to deter them from returning. Clean kitchen surfaces, including walls and ceilings, with a solution of ¼ cup chlorine bleach diluted in 1 gallon of water to remove the cockroach allergen. Neither method, however, will kill the bugs.

Prevention is always your best bet since complete elimination of cockroaches is difficult. Once they've reached the infestation stage, nothing but extermination can help, according to Daniel Hamilos, M.D.

Pesticides are not only environmentally unfriendly but they can agitate respiratory problems. What's worse is that the chemical approach isn't necessarily effective. If you spray your apartment, they will run to the apartment next door, says Dr. Hamilos. Then, when the chemicals have dissipated, they may come back (unless you convince your neighbors to spray, too).

Ultimately, the best thing you can do is to go on a dedicated crumb-and-leak patrol to discourage them in the first place.

> **—Daniel Hamilos, M.D.,** *is an associate professor of medicine at the Washington University School of Medicine and at the Barnes-Jewish Hospital, both in St. Louis, Missouri.*

DEFOREST YOUR HOME

If you're sensitive to mold or pollen, say goodbye to houseplants and ask for chocolate, not roses, on Valentine's Day.

The problem with houseplants is not with the plant itself but with mold in the soil, explains allergist Stuart H. Young, M.D. Flowering plants and cut flowers can also deliver trouble. Although they don't commonly pollinate through the air, some flower pollen can become airborne. In some people, even smelling flowers—especially roses—causes an allergic reaction.

"If you're sensitive to pollen or mold, I wouldn't recommend having any plants or flowers in the house," says Dr. Young. Even the alternatives have their drawbacks: Cacti harbor mold in their soil, and dried flowers and artificial plants collect dust.

"In principle, mold, pollen, and dust should be avoided,"

says Dr. Young, "but we're also dealing with quality of life." Unless you have asthmatic complications connected with your allergy, it's usually just a matter of discomfort. Therefore, if you receive a dozen red roses, the sneezes may be worth it.

—**Stuart H. Young, M.D.,** *is the director of Allergy Fellow's Clinical Education in the department of internal medicine at Mount Sinai Medical Center in New York City and coauthor of* Allergies: The Complete Guide to Diagnosis, Treatment, and Daily Management.

DEMAND A HEALTHY BUILDING

Making sure that the building where you work is up to standards will help you work in peace.

Offices today are fairly self-contained environments due to heating, ventilation, and air-conditioning (HVAC) systems, so you're not going to get a lot of dust mite or mold growth if they're maintained properly. But if the system isn't functioning properly, if there has been water damage in the building, or if the relative humidity is over 55 percent, there is a probability that dust mites and mold are living and growing in your office.

If you suspect that there is a problem, Anthony R. Rooklin, M.D., suggests having the building engineer check the HVAC system to make sure that it is free of organic material and water, which encourage dust mite and mold growth. The system should also be turning over air at an appropriate rate, otherwise allergens will continue to recirculate through the ventilation. This is a good time to check to see if the system has a HEPA (high-efficiency particulate air) filter, which is extremely effective at removing airborne allergens. If not, request that one be installed.

Carpeting, padding, and upholstered furniture are impossible to clean completely even under the best conditions. When they have been damaged by water or kept in a humid environment, you can be sure that mold and dust mite numbers have skyrocketed. If this is a problem, suggest an office redecorating plan using hardwood, vinyl, or tile floors and wood, plastic, or leather furniture.

—Anthony R. Rooklin, M.D., *is a clinical associate professor at the Thomas Jefferson University Hospital in Philadelphia and codirector of the division of allergy and clinical immunology at Crozer Chester Medical Center in Upland, Pennsylvania.*

CLEAR YOUR DESK TO CLEAR THE AIR

A neat desk doesn't just look professional, it holds fewer allergens, too.

Here's another good reason to finally get to that office overhaul you've been talking about: Those piles of papers, invoices, invitations, reports, and last week's lunch tray hold mold, dust, and mites that can add to your allergy problem.

"Clutter is a common workplace problem for people with allergies," according to Gary Weinstock, M.D. Every time you move a piece of paper from one pile to another, a cloud of dust is released into the air for you to inhale. Besides paper, picture frames, knickknacks, little stuffed animals, and other decorations are all dust magnets.

If you must be surrounded by photographs of your loved ones or if you must display your bowling trophy, use a damp cloth to wipe the dust off these objects every week as well as all of the other surfaces around you. And remember that live plants harbor mold in their soil, so you might consider getting rid of the greenery in the office.

Don't toss food into the garbage can by your desk, adds Dr. Weinstock, since mold will begin dining on your leftovers.

—**Gary Weinstock, M.D.,** *is an allergist in Great Neck, New York.*

FILTER OUT OFFICE IMPURITIES

Just because you go out of your way to avoid dogs and pollen, your coworkers don't necessarily do the same. An air purifier can protect you from the allergens others bring into your work space.

You're not a smoker, and you gave up your cat. But a coworker who does smoke or who does have a pet will bring these allergens into the office on his clothing and hair every day. Then there is the wreath on your manager's door that makes your eyes water and the irritatingly sweet potpourri vase in cubicle #12.

Depending on the size of your office and your sensitivity, an air purifier with a HEPA (high-efficiency particulate air) filter can be an effective solution, says Anthony R. Rooklin, M.D.

An air purifier might be helpful at removing allergens like cat and dog dander, irritating odors, and cigarette smoke from the area immediately around your desk. But Dr. Rooklin cautions that there are limitations as to how much it can help. For example, dust mite allergens may settle in the carpet and upholstery, which is beyond an air purifier's scope.

If you decide to purchase an air purifier, bypass the cheap ones at the drugstore and invest in a heavy-duty model with a HEPA filter, sold by one of the many companies specializing in allergy and asthma products. Take into account the size of the area that you want to treat as well as the unit's noise level.

—Anthony R. Rooklin, M.D., *is a clinical associate professor at the Thomas Jefferson University Hospital in Philadelphia and codirector of the division of allergy and clinical immunology at Crozer Cester Medical Center in Upland, Pennsylvania.*

DEFENSIVE DRIVING FOR ALLERGIES

Make car trips sneeze-free affairs by keeping out pollen, dust, and mold spores.

Your mom may have told you that when there is a lightening storm, the car is one of the safest places to be. But if allergies are what you're trying to dodge, the automobile is no haven, especially if you don't clean it out regularly.

"Air-conditioning and fan filters aren't particularly efficient, but they'll still prevent the majority of pollen and mold spores from coming inside if you keep the windows up," says Gary Weinstock, M.D.

Vacuum the inside of your car using a HEPA (high-efficiency particulate air) filter, and toss out all of the dust-gathering, mold-producing clutter stuck under the seat. Remove dust catchers like rearview mirror toys and paper. Clean up food spills that attract insects and mold, or better yet, don't eat in your car at all.

When shopping for a car, a vinyl or leather interior is better than upholstery, because they are easier to clean and dust mites and mold can't invade. "You can steam clean the inside of your car, but that will have a limited ability to get the allergens out," says Dr. Weinstock.

If you are allergic to animals, don't take them for a ride in your car, since their dander will remain long after they have gone.

—**Gary Weinstock, M.D.,** *is an allergist in Great Neck, New York.*

UNDECK YOUR HALLS

'Tis the season for sneezing if you deck your home with allergenic holiday decorations.

Candles, Christmas trees, and roaring fires are signs of a holiday season for many people. But for some people with allergies, they are the harbingers of a sneeze and sniffle season. Before you start decorating, consider some of the potential allergens that can put a damper on the festivities.

"If people are allergic to coniferous trees, I suggest they use artificial trees instead," says Andrew Brown, M.D. Whether you are using an artificial tree or a live one, it's a good idea to spray it outside with a hose before decorating it in order to remove either dust or pollen and molds. Spraying also removes allergens from boughs and swags. And don't neglect to dust ornaments and decorations as well as launder any seasonal textiles like runners and tablecloths.

As for the Yule log, there could be mold in the wood if it's been outside, says Dr. Brown. To reduce the amount of mold exposure, don't bring firewood into your home until you are ready to burn it.

Scented candles can also be a problem, so light up the season with unscented ones if you or your guests have a chemical sensitivity.

—Andrew Brown, M.D., *is an allergist in Gadsden, Alabama.*

SMOKE-FREE IS THE ONLY PLACE TO BE

No ifs, ands, or buts. Allergists say there's absolutely no place for smoking in a healthy house.

If there are smokers in the home, they're doing a lot more harm than just increasing their own health risks. They are producing an allergen that can give others headaches and make it hard for them to breathe. There's also the eye-opening fact that passive smoke increases the likelihood that a child will develop allergies or asthma if he is continually exposed to it during his first 3 to 4 years, says Stuart H. Young, M.D.

Quarantining the smokers to a single room is not the answer. Most homes are not built tightly enough to prevent smoke from seeping out from around door jams and through ventilation systems, says Dr. Young. "An air cleaner will help a little bit, but it's much healthier to banish the smokers outside and away from the house."

Just make sure that they are not out there puffing under someone's window.

—**Stuart H. Young, M.D.,** *is the director of Allergy Fellow's Clinical Education in the department of internal medicine at Mount Sinai Medical Center in New York City and coauthor of* Allergies: The Complete Guide to Diagnosis, Treatment, and Daily Management.

TRY MOTHER NATURE'S AIR FILTERS

Greens make air clean: They're not for everyone, but research shows that certain houseplants can filter away certain allergens and irritants.

As long as you don't have an allergy to the mold that grows in soil and as long as you frequently wash the dust from the leaves, certain houseplants can be very helpful to allergy sufferers, says Valerie Cooksley, R.N.

Research conducted by NASA identified a number of house plants that can work to clean and revitalize the air. The plants filter many allergens and pollutants from the air, including benzene, carbon monoxide, formaldehyde, and trichloroethylene. They also emit a substance that reduces airborne levels of mold spores and bacteria. Lab tests measuring toxic levels of specific chemicals in the air confirmed that the plants listed below are capable of "digesting" such toxins.

If you aren't allergic to the mold, place the following plants in your home and office. One or two plants are all that is needed for every 100 square feet, says Cooksley. Most nurseries will carry these common plants.

- Arneca palm
- Arrowhead vine
- Boston fern
- Dwarf date palm
- English ivy
- Golden pathos
- Peace lily
- Spider plant
- Striped dracaena

—Valerie Cooksley, R.N., *is an aromatherapist and a cofounder of the Institute of Integrative Aromatherapy, which provides aromatherapy education to health care professionals, and the author of* Aromatherapy: A Lifetime Guide to Healing with Essential Oils.

LAUNDER WITH EUCALYPTUS OIL

When you wash sheets and blankets with eucalyptus oil, you wash away those pesky, allergy-provoking dust mites.

Australian researchers found that laundering a wool blanket with eucalyptus oil slashed the dust mite population in the blanket by 95 percent. Along with their extermination properties, essential oils will make your clothes smell great, says Valerie Cooksley, R.N.

For a full load, mix 5 to 10 drops of essential oil of eucalyptus with your favorite liquid (not powder) clothes detergent. You may prefer the eucalyptus citriodora variety because it has a wonderful lemon scent—a nicer aroma than the other varieties of the oil, Cooksley adds. If you prefer, tea tree oil also works.

Use the regular wash cycle, with hot water if your clothes can take it. To give those mites a double whammy, use an automatic dryer on the hottest setting that is safe for your clothes. When you put your clothes in the dryer, you can add a clean, wet washcloth with 5 drops of eucalyptus or tea tree oil. Both oils are available in health food stores or through aromatherapy catalogs.

—**Valerie Cooksley, R.N.,** *is an aromatherapist and a cofounder of the Institute of Integrative Aromatherapy, which provides aromatherapy education to health care professionals, and the author of* Aromatherapy: A Lifetime Guide to Healing with Essential Oils.

Milk Makes Mucus, Fish Fights Inflammation

"Expecting your body to make a well-orchestrated immune response without vital nutrients is like trying to start your car without spark plugs."

—Kenneth Bock, M.D.,
clinical instructor in the department of family medicine at Albany Medical College; founder and director of the Rhinebeck Health Center and the Center for Progressive Medicine in Albany, New York; and coauthor of The Road to Immunity

CONSIDER CUTTING OUT DAIRY

Avoid milk and other dairy products, and you might avoid your allergic rhinitis symptoms, too.

When someone is suffering from allergic rhinitis, the first thing I do is ask them to eliminate dairy products. Very often their allergy symptoms clear immediately, and there is nothing more we need to do." says Michael Traub, N.D.

"Each person has a finite ability to deal with stress, and each allergen is a stress factor," says Dr. Traub. "It's like putting water in a bucket—each allergen will fill the bucket a little more. You are fine until the bucket becomes full. When it overflows, symptoms appear. If dairy is one of your triggers, eliminating it can make a big difference in reducing your total allergic load."

Dairy is both the most common food allergy (along with wheat) and very easy to avoid, compared to airborne allergens. So heed Dr. Traub's advice. For 6 weeks, cut out all dairy products from your diet. In the meantime, try melted soy cheese on your sandwiches and homemade pizza. Use soy or rice milk in place of cow's milk.

When the 6 weeks are up, try dairy again. If in fact you are allergic, you'll notice it right away. The symptoms are usually a runny nose and extra mucus. You may even feel tired, achy, or sneezy within 24 to 72 hours after eating dairy. If so, keep your allergy load lighter by regularly staying off milk products.

Approximately 25 percent or more of people with airborne allergies also have a milk allergy. But even if you don't have the classic symptoms, you may still want to avoid milk because it creates extra mucus in your body, contributing to congestion and respiratory distress, Dr. Traub says.

> **—Michael Traub, N.D.,** *is a naturopathic doctor in Kailua Kona, Hawaii, and a staff member of North Hawaii Community Hospital in Kamuela.*

COOK YOUR ENEMIES

Some people with pollen allergies get what's called a cross-reaction when they eat certain raw fruits and vegetables. Beat the cycle by cooking these problem foods.

No one knows exactly why people with pollen allergies cross-react to certain produce, but it happens. Fortunately, these cross-reactions are avoidable.

If you have cross-reactions to certain fruits or vegetables, you'll know because you get itching in the mouth, face, and throat. Unlike the dangers associated with actual food allergies, cross-reactions—however unpleasant—are certainly not life threatening, says Steve L. Taylor, Ph.D.

The solution is this simple: Cook the offending produce instead of eating it raw. If your allergy is seasonal, then you only need to cook or avoid your offending food at that time. For example, people with a birch tree pollen allergy often cross-react with fresh apples, peaches, pears, and cherries. So they need to cook the offending fruits until the allergy season has passed. Then, they can enjoy them again fresh in January, when the birch tree pollen is dormant.

In the meantime, you may not get to crunch your way

through apple skins, but you can still enjoy apple pie, cherry cobbler, hot cider, and spicy applesauce. As long as the fruit is exposed to enough heat, cooking will destroy the allergen. You also can pop the top on canned pears or peaches because the canning process uses high heat to preserve food.

People with the very common mugwort pollen allergy often cross-react with raw celery. "You'll have no problem eating celery seed or cooked celery," says Dr. Taylor, "but fresh celery may cause a mild itching problem."

The most common cross-reaction? People who sneeze and get runny noses around ragweed may also have a problem with fresh melons. Although most people don't eat warm or canned melons, you can enjoy other fresh fruit until the allergy season passes.

> **—Steve L. Taylor, Ph.D.,** *is the department head and a professor of food science and technology at the University of Nebraska in Lincoln.*

FISH FOR SMARTER FATS

If you have respiratory problems, first change your diet to include less processed food. Then eat more fish or take fish oil in capsule form.

Twenty-one to 65 percent of allergic rhinitis sufferers also have asthma. The two conditions are so often found together that Canadian researchers termed the combination *allergic rhinobronchitis.* One way to take control of allergic rhinobronchitis is by modifying your diet.

K. Shane Broughton, Ph.D., suggests that changing the kind of fat you eat might decrease your breathing problems, as it did for half the people in his University of Wyoming study. Nineteen people with asthma took breathing tests. They were then treated with fish oil capsules daily for a month during allergy season. Thirty days later, a retest showed that half of the people were breathing easier—far more than the people in a control group who weren't taking any fish oil.

Many people eat too much of the omega-6 fatty acids (found in vegetable oils, margarine, potato chips, French fries, and processed foods) and not enough of the omega-3 fatty acids (found in oily fish like salmon, herring, sardines, and anchovies), says Dr. Broughton. It's that imbalance that may partially account for the asthma problem.

So get back in balance by taking in fewer fries and cookies—which are high in omega-6—and more fish or fish oil, with it's omega-3 benefits.

Subjects in Dr. Broughton's study got results with 7 fish oil capsules at bedtime for at least a month. Each capsule contained 1 gram of fat, half of that from omega-3 fatty acids. Be sure to take fish oil, not fish-liver oil, which is toxic in high amounts.

Do not take fish oil capsules if you have a bleeding disorder or high blood pressure; if you take blood thinning medication regularly, including aspirin; or if you are allergic to any kind of fish. People with diabetes should not take fish oil because of its high fat content.

—K. Shane Broughton, Ph.D., *is an associate professor of nutrition at the University of Wyoming in Laramie.*

TAKE MAGNESIUM FOR EASIER BREATHING

Hay fever is commonly accompanied by asthmatic wheezing. If you have trouble catching your breath, magnesium may smooth out the problem.

During an asthma attack, the muscles in your chest tighten and your airways narrow, making each breath a struggle. That's why the mineral magnesium, which is known to relax the smooth walls of the muscles and stop spasms, is recommended.

Kendall Gerdes, M.D., says that for maximum relief you should take as much magnesium as your body can handle. "The tolerable range is different for everyone. Some people are sensitive to 100 milligrams a day while others can take 1,000 milligrams twice a day," explains Dr. Gerdes. Your body will signal you to cut back when you get diarrhea.

Dr. Gerdes suggests starting out with the dosage of 100 milligrams of an easily absorbable form of magnesium, like magnesium gluconate, twice a day, for 2 days. If you don't experience intestinal upset, add 100 milligrams to your dosage. If you still have a tight chest, continue to double the dosage every 2 days until you start to have loose stools. Go back to the previous dose, which is your maximum tolerable amount, and stay on it.

People with heart or kidney problems should check with their doctors before taking supplemental magnesium. And be sure to talk to your doctor about supplemental magnesium if you get diarrhea as soon as you start taking it.

—Kendall Gerdes, M.D., *is an allergist and the director of Environmental Medicine Associates in Denver.*

BE SMART AT BARBECUES

Theophylline can be a big help in controlling allergy-complicated asthma symptoms. But eating high-protein and grilled foods can cause your body to lose this needed medicine.

If your pollen allergies are complicated by asthma, you may be prescribed the bronchodilator theophylline (Slo-Bid, Slo-Phyllin, Theo-Dur). If so, outdoor barbecue parties featuring large slabs of charcoal-grilled meat and mounds of coleslaw and broccoli salad must be celebrated sensibly.

Diet has a huge impact on how fast your body metabolizes theophylline, says Chris Meletis, N.D. When you eat big portions of meat, chicken, and fish, theophylline quickly rushes out of your body. Charcoal grilling makes the problem worse. In fact, charcoal is so good at absorbing theophylline that it is used to cure life-threatening theophylline overdoses.

In addition, the cabbage in your coleslaw—as well as other cruciferous vegetables like broccoli, cauliflower, kale, and Brussels sprouts—increases the problem of theophylline loss.

The best approach for maintaining proper theophylline levels is to eat consistent amounts of protein and carbohydrates, and avoid charcoal-grilled foods.

—Chris Meletis, N.D., *is the dean of clinical affairs at the National College of Naturopathic Medicine in Portland, Oregon.*

TRY MSM, THE BREAKTHROUGH SUPPLEMENT

Build your resistance to sniffles and sneezes by taking a sulfur compound.

Chemists may know it as methsulfonyl methane, a high-sulfur metabolite of dimethyl sulfoxide, but many people with allergies know MSM as an anti-inflammatory that shows great promise in preventing allergy and asthma symptoms.

Unlike vitamin C, an antihistamine that reduces symptoms *after* they have begun, MSM stabilizes cell membranes so they're more resistant to releasing the histamine that causes your allergic reactions in the first place, according to Chris Meletis, N.D.

MSM occurs naturally in fruits and vegetables, but you can buy it in capsule form at health food stores. "For most adults, a dose of 500 to 1,000 milligrams three times a day with meals works well," says Dr. Meletis. If you have gastrointestinal upset, decrease the amount.

Since it hasn't been well-tested on pregnant women, he does not recommend MSM for pregnant or lactating women. Dr. Meletis also cautions that you shouldn't take MSM if you have a history of reacting badly to sulfur compounds. For most other people, it's safe, he says.

—Chris Meletis, N.D., *is the dean of clinical affairs at the National College of Naturopathic Medicine in Portland, Oregon.*

MAKE SOME CHICKEN SOUP WITH A KICK

A properly made chicken soup can clear away most of your allergy symptoms. Making it extra pungent, hot, and peppery will kick up the healing power of this classic remedy even higher.

Chicken soup has been used as a symptomatic remedy for congestion for more than 800 years. In his recipe, Irwin Ziment, M.D., enhanced the healing ingredients to get maximum relief.

To begin with, chicken skin is rich in cysteine, an antioxidant amino acid that loosens mucus, he says. Pepper will help clear your nose. Garlic stimulates receptors in your mouth, tongue, throat, and stomach to cause an outpouring of watery fluid to dilute sticky secretions and make them easier to remove by coughing. If any infections are developing from your chronic allergic congestion, the garlic and the onions can offer antibacterial and antiviral support.

"It's powerful stuff—more like a drug than a soup," says Dr. Ziment. Until you get used to it, you may need to sip it in very small doses. But take at least 1 teaspoon to 4 tablespoons at a time, three or four times a day, to have an effect.

Stay nearby while the soup simmers, and inhale the fumes that rise from the pot. Inhalation is part of the healing recipe, he says.

Dr. Ziment's Kickin' Chicken Soup

1   chicken (2½ to 3 pounds), cut into pieces
2   cans low-sodium chicken broth (or 3½ cups
     homemade stock)
1   garlic head (about 15 cloves)
1   medium onion, quartered
3   celery rib, chopped
½   pound carrots, peeled and coarsely chopped
1   teaspoon dried basil
     pepper (as much as you can take)

Place chicken pieces, with skin and bones, in a large pot. Add the broth or stock and enough water to cover the chicken pieces. Simmer the chicken for about 1 hour, or until tender.

Remove the chicken and allow to cool. When cool enough to touch, remove and discard the skin and bones. Coarsely chop the chicken and return it to the pot.

Add the garlic, onion, celery, carrots, basil, and pepper. Add enough water to cover the vegetables, then simmer 20 to 30 minutes, or until the vegetables are tender.

Makes 4 to 6 servings.

Pressed for time? Sprinkle pepper, curry powder, and garlic into canned chicken broth. Heat to simmering, then sip. Don't forget to inhale over the pot while it's warming.

—Irwin Ziment, M.D., *is a pulmonary specialist at the Olive View–UCLA Medical Center in Sylmar, California.*

DON'T TAKE YOUR ALLERGY MEDICINE WITH GRAPEFRUIT JUICE

Allergy medicine can have some pretty unpleasant side effects. Making the mistake of taking it with grapefruit juice could shoot the drug's effects into the danger zone.

Washing down your prescription allergy medicine such as fexofenadine (Allegra), loratadine (Claritin), or astemizole (Hismana) with grapefruit juice could increase blood levels of these anti-allergy medications and possibly their side effects as well.

The reason? Unlike other fruit juices, grapefruit contains high levels of the bioflavonoid, naringin, which appears to allow more of certain drugs (at least 20 have been tested so far) to be absorbed into your bloodstream. That means you might get the effects of a bigger dose, even when you take the standard amount. Side effects like drowsiness or excitability may increase, explains Chris Meletis, N.D.

A study by the London Health Sciences Center in Ontario, showed that the effect of a single glass of grapefruit juice could last 24 hours, suggesting that several glasses a day could have a cumulative effect. And a study by the University of Helsinki, Finland, showed that drinking the equivalent of 5 cups of grapefruit juice a day for 2 consecutive days affected the actual dose of one drug for up to 72 hours.

While there are no reported studies specifically on interactions between grapefruit and allergy medication, until we know more, stick with water, recommends Dr. Meletis.

—Chris Meletis, N.D., *is the dean of clinical affairs at the National College of Naturopathic Medicine in Portland, Oregon.*

CLEAR UP
WITH HORSERADISH

Relieving stuffed sinuses can be as simple as drinking a Russian tonic or ordering the right condiment with your sushi.

When allergies have you congested, grate some horse-radish root. The root of this plant in the cabbage family works somewhat like tear gas, making your eyes water and nose run, thereby clearing up mucus.

"Take it like the Russians do," says Irwin Ziment, M.D. "That's drinking 1 teaspoon of freshly grated horseradish in a glass of warm water with a teaspoon of honey."

If you're apprehensive about swallowing the pungent root, another option is to use it as a gargle. Either way, the honey makes the horseradish stick to the back of your throat and, by reflex, stimulates your nose and lungs to produce more mucus. By spitting and blowing your nose, you expel the mucus.

You can also get the extra-hot condiment called wasabi that's served at Japanese restaurants. The potent green horseradish-like sauce is superb for cleaning out your nose and sinuses. But don't start by mounding it on your next dragon roll. The tolerance varies from person to person. "If you're not used to it, you're in for a real shock, so start with a small amount," warns Dr. Ziment.

In fact, don't eat horseradish or wasabi at all if you have stomach inflammation problems or kidney disorders.

—Irwin Ziment, M.D., *is a pulmonary specialist at the Olive View–UCLA Medical Center in Sylmar, California.*

WEIGH YOUR LIQUID ASSETS

Your allergy and hay fever medications may temporarily relieve your runny nose and watery eyes, but be careful how much you let yourself dry up. If you're on allergy medicine, know the signals of dehydration.

Water, water, everywhere. . . and you need even more water than the traditional eight glasses a day when your pollen allergies are at their peak. Getting enough fluid helps break down phlegm and dilute mucus. The problem is that many of the medications that dry up your sinuses and runny nose also dry up all of your other body fluids.

"Use your scale as your guide," says Tammy Baker, R.D., who wrestles with seasonal allergies. "Two cups of water weighs 1 pound. If you take an allergy pill and suddenly lose a couple of pounds, you're dehydrated and need to drink enough extra fluids (in this case, 4 cups) to get back to normal." Dark-colored urine is another sign that you need more liquids.

Just 2 percent dehydration (losing as little as 2½ pounds in a 120-pound woman) can cause headache, fatigue, loss of appetite, flushed skin, heat intolerance, light-headedness, dry mouth and eyes, and a burning sensation in the stomach.

Besides water, a good source of fluid is fruits and vegetables because they are 80 to 90 percent water.

For suggestions on how to remember to drink enough water every day, see page 105.

—Tammy Baker, R.D., *is a Phoenix-based spokesperson for the American Dietetic Association.*

LET CHILIES SPICE OUT YOUR CONGESTION

While it wakes up your palate, spicy Mexican food can also help clear your nasal passages.

It's hard to breathe and eat at the same time when your allergies have you stuffed up, which causes you to miss out on the gastronomic joy of subtle flavors. But by adding a flavoring agent that's nothing close to subtle, you can clear up the problem. Introducing chile peppers into your food can break through just about any case of congestion.

The active ingredient in chile peppers comes from capsaicin, the chemical that lends the fiery taste, makes your eyes water and nose run, and triggers the brain to produce endorphins, which are natural painkillers that promote a sense of well-being and stimulation.

Capsaicin survives cooking and freezing, and it is also

active in powder form—so long as the powder still clumps up in the container, signaling that the natural oils have not evaporated.

The easiest way to get chile peppers into your diet when you're feeling out-of-sorts is to add salsa to low-fat Mexican food. You can also shake crushed red pepper (which is actually chile peppers) into soups and stews and onto eggs. Or try jalapeño peppers. "They're relatively mild peppers and taste great with almost everything," says Tammy Baker, R.D. "Try adding some slices to sandwiches."

—**Tammy Baker, R.D.,** *is a Phoenix-based spokesperson for the American Dietetic Association.*

TAKE A QUERCETIN COCKTAIL

This wonderful supplement can either prevent an allergy attack or stop one in its tracks. Either way, combine it with other supplements for maximum effect.

Quercetin is a bioflavonoid that stabilizes the immune system cells that release histamine, a trigger for some of your worst allergic reactions like runny nose and burning eyes. "I take a daily quercetin complex year-round to prevent allergic rhinitis," says Sandra Pinkham, M.D.

The complex she recommends (and takes herself) contains 330 milligrams of quercetin, 200 milligrams of vitamin C, 13 milligrams of magnesium, and 100 milligrams of bromelain, an anti-inflammatory agent in pineapple. The combination is important because quercetin alone is not well-absorbed.

"The preventive approach is best," Dr. Pinkham emphasizes. So as allergy season blooms, she recommends increasing the quercetin complex to three times a day, along with an additional 1,000 milligrams of buffered vitamin C powder three times a day, and a 5-milligram chewable zinc tablet three or four times a day.

But for urgent relief, especially at night, a combination of 1,000 milligrams of vitamin C, 5 milligrams of chewable zinc, the quercetin complex, and 2 deglycyrrhizinated licorice tablets works wonders. "In about 15 minutes, I can breathe easy again," Dr. Pinkham says.

Just be aware that excess vitamin C may cause diarrhea in some people, so you will need to cut back the amount if you have loose stools. Do not take bromelain if you are allergic to pineapple or if you regularly take aspirin or anticoagulants (blood thinners). Licorice should be avoided if you have liver or kidney disorders, diabetes, or high blood pressure—and it shouldn't be used regularly by anyone for more than 6 weeks.

—Sandra Pinkham, M.D., *is a physician in Columbus, Ohio.*

KNOW YOUR A'S, B'S, AND D'S

Vitamins can be powerful natural prescriptions for relief.

When you're using nutrition to fight allergic rhinitis, you need an array of nutrients that help tissues function more effectively. You may need to try different combinations to see what is most effective for you, but here are some general guidelines offered by Sandra Pinkham, M.D.

Patients who are coughing and sneezing or are very stressed out can take 500 milligrams of the anti-inflammatory pantothenic acid two or three times a day. Pantothenic acid supports the adrenal glands in producing cortisol, which reduces congestion. You can get it as part of an inexpensive vitamin B complex.

"I also recommend a multivitamin that contains 700 IU of vitamin D and at least 5,000 but not more than 10,000 IU of preformed vitamin A (that's true vitamin A and not beta-carotene)," adds Dr. Pinkham. Both vitamin A and vitamin D benefit the moist tissues that line the mouth, nose, and throat by enabling them to act as an effective barrier against invading organisms.

—**Sandra Pinkham, M.D.,** *is a physician in Columbus, Ohio.*

CONSUME QUERCETIN-RICH FOODS

Upping your fruits and vegetables will be a real bonus to getting this natural antihistamine.

Quercetin, a bioflavonoid recommended to prevent allergic rhinitis, is found naturally in onions, kale, leaf lettuce, cranberries, tea, wine, apples, buckwheat, and citrus fruit.

Yellow onions are the richest quercetin source, which is good news, since adding onions makes almost any dish taste better, according to chef-trained registered dietitian Barbara Gollman. Mound raw onions onto sandwiches, toss them into salads, or chop them into salsa or gazpacho. And quercetin survives cooking, so you can simmer up a big batch of onion soup, add extra onions to stews, or sauté a chopped onion in olive oil to serve over chicken or fish.

Buckwheat, another quercetin-rich food, is the fruit of a plant related to rhubarb, with an intense nutty flavor. Because it's higher in protein than grains, it's an excellent food for vegetarians and people with allergies. Enjoy buckwheat pancakes or a dinner side dish of dark, coarsely ground groats called kasha. Buckwheat flour contains no gluten (it actually has no relation to wheat), so it can't be used by itself for baking. You can substitute it, however, for one-quarter to one-half of the wheat flour in most recipes.

—Barbara Gollman, R.D., *is a consulting dietitian, nutrition educator, and culinary arts expert in Dallas and author of* The Phytopia Cookbook.

GET ACQUAINTED WITH KALE

Although kale is loaded with histamine-beating quercetin, few people know how to serve it. Here's a tasty way to get acquainted.

Some people slink dubiously past the gigantic green leaves sticking out of the produce aisle between the Brussels sprouts and spinach. Many people who have never tasted kale have already decided that they don't like this strange-looking vegetable and prefer to relegate it to the realm of salad-bar garnish.

But even for the ones who are curious, remarks Barbara Gollman, R.D., who knows what to do with it?

To get people on friendlier terms with this nutrient-rich leaf, Gollman created this zesty "phytopia pesto." You can pour it over pasta, pile it on bruschetta, or spread it on sandwiches and quesadillas. No one will ever guess that it's kale—until their allergy symptoms start disappearing.

Phytopia Pesto

¾   pound kale, washed, stemmed, and coarsely chopped
3–4 garlic cloves, peeled
1   cup fresh basil leaves, washed and stemmed
    juice of 1 lemon
2   tablespoons extra-virgin olive oil
1   teaspoon salt
    freshly ground black pepper, to taste

Place the kale in a large microwaveable bowl and cover. Microwave on high power for 5 minutes. Stir and microwave for another 5 minutes. Let stand 2 to 3 minutes, then remove cover to cool.

Drop garlic into the bowl of a food processor with the motor running. When finely minced, add the basil and cooked kale. Process until uniform.

Add the lemon juice, oil, salt, and pepper. Serve as you would pesto.

Makes 4 servings.

—Barbara Gollman, R.D., *is a consulting dietitian, nutrition educator, and culinary arts expert in Dallas and author of* The Phytopia Cookbook.

TRY THE "MASTER CLEANSER"

Consuming nothing but this energizing tonic for a few days could truly clear out your symptoms for good.

Natural health doctors often attribute allergy susceptibility to toxins—unhealthy contaminants in your body—and a sluggish digestive system. Elson Haas, M.D., had allergies before he took care of them through fasting on juice and eating a healthier diet.

"Fifteen years ago, I had allergic rhinitis. By the third day of my juice cleansing, my head was clear; and I stayed clear for years," says Dr. Haas.

In Dr. Haas's healing tonic, everyday ingredients play a medicinal role. The lemon or lime juice serves as an astringent that breaks up fats and constricts the tissues in your respiratory system to clear mucus and toxins. Maple syrup will keep your blood sugar level up, so you are energetic while you fast. The ground red pepper is both a natural stimulant and a diuretic, which creates the important flushing action. The water itself is also a natural cleanser.

Dr. Haas's Detox Tonic

2 tablespoons freshly squeezed lemon or lime juice
1 tablespoon pure maple syrup
   dash of ground red pepper
8 ounces water

Stir the lemon or lime juice, syrup, and pepper into the water.

Drink 1 or 2 glasses every 2 hours, especially if you feel hungry or low on energy, for a total of 8 to 12 glasses a day. Be sure to rinse your mouth with water each time to protect your teeth from the citrus acidity.

For maximum cleansing, says Dr. Haas, you need to be sure your bowels are moving. "Start every *other* morning by drinking 2 teaspoons of sea salt dissolved in 2 quarts of warm water," he says. If you're salt sensitive, use an herbal laxative instead.

Check with your doctor before beginning a fast. Healthy people can usually fast safely for 1 to 3 days at a time for a total of 10 days a year. Fasting should be done during a time of rest. For example, try doing it on a weekend. Ease into your fast by eliminating heavy foods like proteins, starches, and sugars; and start eating fresh fruits and vegetables a few days before. Then start fasting Friday morning and continue until Sunday at dinnertime, easing back into the work week with a small meal of fruit. Be sure to drink plenty of water during your fast and avoid acetaminophen, which is too much of a burden on your liver during a fast.

Fasting is not for everyone, Dr. Haas warns. Pregnant or lactating women, people who are very fatigued or nutritionally deficient or very sick should not use this fast. If you have a chronic illness, use the fast only under your physician's guidance.

—**Elson Haas, M.D.,** *is the medical director and founder of the Preventive Medical Center of Marin in San Rafael, California, and author of* Staying Healthy with Nutrition.

CHOOSE CHOLAGOGUES

The root of your allergic respiratory
problems could be your digestion.
Therefore, stimulating your
gallbladder and liver could help
you withstand allergies.

Based on the traditional herbalism premise that upper respiratory problems are aggravated by a heavy or sluggish digestion, Lisa Meserole, N.D., recommends eating from the category of foods herbalists call cholagogues. "*Cholagogue* is a term for foods and herbs that act as gallbladder and liver stimulants," she says.

Cholagogue vegetables include beets, artichokes, the burdock root used in Asian cooking, and bitter greens—like European endive, arugula, and cilantro. Some fruits will also help with sluggish bile acid secretion, but they vary from person to person. The ones most likely to work, says Dr. Meserole, are apples, pears, and some berries. The spice turmeric, which makes the yellow color in curry powder, is also a cholagogue.

These foods spur your gallbladder to contract and squirt bile into your upper gut. Bile is what's known as an emulsifier, which makes fat more digestible and neutralizes the acidic, partially digested food in your stomach. In addition, bile's high salt content draws water into the gut, stimulating peristalsis, so contents move along.

People who have gallstones or bile duct blockage should avoid cholagogues, since stimulating gallbladder contractions could cause gallstones to become impacted, Dr. Meserole cautions.

—Lisa Meserole, N.D., *is a research consultant and faculty member at Bastyr University and a naturopathic physician at Healing Arts in Seattle.*

BUZZ AWAY ALLERGIES

Eat like a bee and become allergy-free.

Pollen is a nightmare for people with allergies, but you don't see bees sneezing as they fly from one plant to the next. Here's how to build an immunity like a honeybee's.

"I've met many people who claim to have lost pollen allergies by eating local bee pollen every day for a period of months," says Andrew Weil, M.D.

The theory is that allergies are a learned response, and anything that is learned can be unlearned. Eating local pollen is similar to getting an allergy shot, says Dr. Weil, in that you're regularly exposed to the allergen in a small amount until you hopefully learn to tolerate it.

Visit a nearby beekeeper or your local health food store to get local bee pollen, says Dr. Weil. It *has* to be local, he stresses, because you need to start exposing yourself to the specific spectrum of pollens in your area.

"Then, start out by taking only a tiny crumb once a day. Use extreme caution since some people are violently allergic to pollen—so stop eating it entirely if you experience any itching in your throat," says Dr. Weil.

Once you work your way up to a teaspoon a day, continue eating it for several months, until signs of your allergies begin to disappear.

Although it's rare, bee pollen may cause life-threatening anaphylactic shock, so steer clear of it if you have a history of anaphylactic reactions. Stop taking bee pollen if you get stomach pain, diarrhea, itching in the mouth, or other discomforts. If you have asthma or diabetes, check with your doctor before taking bee pollen.

—Andrew Weil, M.D., *is a clinical professor of internal medicine at the University of Arizona School of Medicine in Tucson, the founder and director of the program in integrative medicine, and author of numerous holistic health books, including* 8 Weeks to Optimum Health.

Getting
Natural Relief

"Alternative therapies for allergies have one common goal: to bring your body into a natural state of balance so that your immune system can function properly. Each remedy attempts to teach your body to heal itself, with help only from natural substances, human touch, and common sense."

—Glenn S. Rothfeld, M.D.,
clinical instructor at Tufts University School of Medicine in Boston; director of the American WholeHealth Center in Arlington, Massachusetts; and author of Natural Medicine for Allergies

TAKE THE STING OUT OF YOUR SYMPTOMS

The herbal remedy stinging nettle can relieve your symptoms and free you from the side effects associated with prescription drugs.

A natural alternative to allergy prescription drugs is the stinging nettle plant. Herbalists and doctors report that allergic rhinitis symptoms go away quickly for most people taking this herbal remedy.

Andrew Weil, M.D., considers stinging nettle a more desirable form of allergy treatment than most pharmaceutical or over-the-counter options. "My main objection to allergy drugs like antihistamines and steroids is that they suppress or block the allergic process and in doing so, only perpetuate the problem," says Dr. Weil.

"I have taught many patients to get off antihistamines and onto stinging nettle with good results," he says. Dr. Weil has suffered intense allergic reactions to ragweed his whole life, and personal experience has taught him that treatment with stinging nettle is more effective than treatment with antihistamines.

When the National College of Naturopathic Medicine in Portland, Oregon, studied the effects of stinging nettle on people with airborne allergies, 58 percent of those taking stinging nettle said they achieved moderate or excellent relief after just 1 week.

Stinging nettle is a common plant throughout the world. You may have brushed by the plant when you walked through a field overgrown with weeds. For allergy relief, you don't have to comb the fields for wild plants. Dr. Weil says the form to use is the freeze-dried leaves, which are sold in capsules at health food stores. In some rare cases, nettle can cause symptoms to worsen, so start with 1 capsule a day for the first 2 days. If your reaction is okay, proceed to Dr. Weil's recommended dosage of 2 capsules every 2 to 4 hours as needed to control symptoms. Typical capsules are 300 milligrams.

> **—Andrew Weil, M.D.,** *is a clinical professor of internal medicine at the University of Arizona School of Medicine in Tucson, the founder and director of the program in integrative medicine, and author of numerous holistic health books, including* 8 Weeks to Optimum Health.

SOAK AWAY ALLERGIES

Add some vitamin C and bubbles to the tub and feel your allergy irritations float away.

Taking a fizzy vitamin C bath is not only relaxing but it also has medicinal effects.

While you soak, some of the vitamin C is absorbed into the skin. Consequently, some of it may get into the bloodstream, where it will help relieve the allergy symptoms of inflammation.

"Vitamin C also makes the water slightly acidic, building a protective layer on your skin to prevent allergens from penetrating into your body—we call it the acid mantle," explains Agatha Thrash, M.D. This protection should last all day—or up to 2 days—if you do not take a shower after the vitamin C bath, says Dr. Thrash.

She recommends adding 3 tablespoons of ascorbic acid powder (available in most health food stores) to a warm bath. This form of vitamin C makes your bath feel like a spa because it has a slight effervescent effect.

—Agatha Thrash, M.D., *is a medical pathologist and the cofounder and codirector of Uchee Pines Institute, a rural natural healing center near Seale, Alabama.*

RESCUE A RUNNY NOSE WITH SOOTHING SAGE TEA

Sage was once so revered by ancient healers that it was considered a tonic that assured people of immortality. Today's herbalists can't promise eternal life, but they do recommend sage to give you a boost when allergies make you miserable.

Because of its drying effect, sage is an excellent remedy for congestion and sniffles, says herbal expert Betzy Bancroft. It can also boost the immune system, which could help prevent allergies from getting worse. Another bonus: Sage can help prevent infections that can result from chronic allergies, such sinusitis and ear infection.

Bancroft recommends a cup of sage tea when your runny nose symptoms occur. It can be taken up to six times a day.

But sage will disappoint you if it's not properly stored. All herbs, including sage tea, should be kept in airtight glass containers and stored in a cool, dark place to retain freshness. When purchasing the tea, make sure it looks and smells fresh.

As tempting as this remedy is, it's not for everyone. Do not use sage if you are pregnant, nursing, hypoglycemic, or undergoing anticonvulsant therapy. Sage can increase the sedative side effects of some drugs.

> **—Betzy Bancroft** *is a professional member of the American Herbalists Guild and manager of Herbalist and Alchemist, a botanical medicine production company and herbalism school in Washington, New Jersey.*

CRADLE YOUR EYES

You already know the comfort from a perfect, cozy pillow under your head. Get a special pillow for your eyes, too, for soothing sore sinuses and helping you to de-stress.

If you place an "eye pillow" over your eyes and forehead when you are trying to fall asleep, the pillow might help relieve your allergy-rankled sinuses, says yoga expert Linda Rado.

Eye pillows look like miniature pillows with a very soft casing (usually silk). But instead of being filled with cotton or foam, eye pillows are usually filled with flaxseed along with soothing herbs like lavender or chamomile. They're available at health food stores or through yoga supply catalogs.

Resting on top of your eyes and forehead, an eye pillow applies light pressure on the brow bone and eyelids, thereby softening the bones of the skull, explains Rado. When your skull expands, the sinus passages soften up. That helps relieve the pressure and enables the sinuses to drain, she says.

The eye pillow also blocks out light and relaxes the facial muscles. This assisted "darkening" helps bring stillness to the active mind by drawing the senses inward, says Rado. The combination of a quiet mind and relaxed facial muscles bring a peaceful state both internally and externally, helpful for overcoming stress-related allergy symptoms.

—Linda Rado, R.Y.T., *is a professional yoga teacher, yoga therapist, and co-owner of The Studio, a yoga center in West Reading, Pennsylvania. Certified in three schools of yoga, she continues advanced studies at Master Yoga Academy in La Jolla, California.*

BATHE YOUR EYES WITH A DROP OF BULGARIAN ROSE WATER

A couple of drops of pure Bulgarian rose water can clear up inflamed and itchy eyes.

Think of how refreshed you feel when you just catch a whiff of rose in the air. The same essence that creates that aroma can also help refresh irritated eyes, according to aromatherapists. That's because rose has anti-inflammatory agents.

Bulgarian rose water is traditionally prescribed by herbalists and aromatherapists to treat conjunctivitis—an infection in the delicate membrane lining the eyelids, often caused by allergies.

"It might sting a little at first," says aromatherapy expert John Steele, "but then there is this marvelous release—your eyes will look clear and feel relieved."

Make sure the rose water is Bulgarian, he says. The rose variety grown in Bulgaria, *Rosa damascena,* has no toxic or irritating effects. Bulgaria is known as the Valley of the Roses because the country has a tradition of making the finest quality rose water in the world, Steele adds.

Steele recommends 1 drop of *Rosa damascena* water in each eye as needed when allergy symptoms irritate your eyes. You can repeat the application up to four times daily. (But you'll need to see a doctor if the redness and irritation don't go away within a couple of days.)

—John Steele *practices at Life Tree Aromatix, an aromatherapy consulting firm in Los Angeles.*

ARREST ALLERGY SYMPTOMS WITH AROMATHERAPY

Essential oils are multibeneficial for the treatment of chronic allergy symptoms.

The essential oils of eucalyptus, German chamomile, and patchouli can help relieve inflammation and boost immunity. They naturally purify the air and encourage deep breathing, says Valerie Cooksley, R.N.

"The oils not only smell good but they are also wonderfully relaxing," says Cooksley. With the antistress properties of essential oils, you may have all you need to help prevent or alleviate an allergy attack.

Cooksley offers a combination that she calls hay fever rescue mix: 3 parts eucalyptus radiata essential oil, 1 part German chamomile essential oil, and 1 part patchouli or sandalwood essential oil.

Put the mixture in a "nonheating" style of diffuser, in which a little electric-powered pump forces air and tiny droplets of your oil into the room. Turn it on (or preset an electronic timer) three, four, or five times a day for 15 minutes. The healing oil will remain suspended in the air for several hours.

Diffusers and essential oils can be purchased at health food stores. Make sure you purchase high-quality, pure essential oils since they will have the most therapeutic effect, Cooksley says.

As a note of caution, don't use this remedy for more than 2 weeks straight without the guidance of a qualified practitioner, and don't use it while you are using homeopathic remedies.

—Valerie Cooksley, R.N., *is an aromatherapist and a cofounder of the Institute of Integrative Aromatherapy, which provides aromatherapy education to health care professionals; and the author of* Aromatherapy: A Lifetime Guide to Healing with Essential Oils.

WARM YOUR FEET FOR ALLERGY RELIEF

Relax your feet—and your allergy symptoms—with a simple footbath.

Medical evidence suggests that immersing your feet in warm water can significantly decrease your allergy symptoms. There is certainly no harm—so why not plunge your dogs in a tub of warm water and sink into a pair of fuzzy bunny slippers the next time your allergies give you nasal problems?

"It's worth a try," says Berrylin J. Ferguson, M.D. "If nothing else, you end up feeling relaxed and comfortably warm. At best, you stop sniffling and sneezing."

In a study performed at the University of Chicago, people with seasonal allergic rhinitis were exposed to three successive, increasing doses of their allergens. Their feet were immersed in warm water or room temperature water for 5 minutes before and during each exposure. Researchers discovered that the people who soaked their feet in warm water had significantly reduced symptoms of allergy compared to those who didn't. Thus, it was concluded that warming the feet decreases allergic nasal symptoms.

In light of the study, Dr. Ferguson says a 5-minute footbath when you are experiencing allergy symptoms may be helpful. Make sure you dry your feet and moisturize them well afterward. She recommends putting on a pair of really warm socks or slippers when you are finished.

There is a good possibility that foot warmers work for the same reason the warm water does, says Dr. Ferguson. In fact, the day may come, she says, when foot warmers are sold at health food stores in the allergy-relief section.

—Berrylin J. Ferguson, M.D., *is an associate professor of otolaryngology and chief of the division of sino-nasal disorders at the University of Pittsburgh in Pennsylvania.*

BUTTER UP TO ALLERGY RELIEF

By applying ghee, otherwise known as clarified butter, to your nose, your chances of getting seasonal allergy symptoms may melt away.

Clarified butter is an ingredient in many Indian foods. But in Ayurvedic medicine—the traditional form of medical care in India—ghee is also used to treat allergies.

"The reason that lubricating the nostrils with ghee, or clarified butter, can help to prevent allergy attacks is because the ghee makes it very difficult for allergens to penetrate the nasal passages," says Vasant Lad, M.A.Sc., B.A.M.S.

To make ghee, melt 2 pounds of unsalted butter in a heavy saucepan over medium heat. As soon as the butter begins to boil and foam, reduce the heat to a simmer. Keep the melted butter at a steady simmer until it is golden in color and no foam remains on top. Whitish curds (the cholesterol) will sink to the bottom. When these curds turn light tan, the ghee is ready. Cool the mixture and strain off the curds with a wire strainer.

This mixture should last for several weeks if you store it on a shelf in a tightly closed jar that was sterilized by boiling it in water or washing it in a dishwasher. Using an eye-dropper or a clean, dry spoon, retrieve 3 drops of the liquid ghee and place it on the tip of your pinky finger. Rub it everywhere inside each nostril, rotating it, as far as it is comfortable. Apply the ghee three times a day—morning, midday, and evening—during the allergy season.

—Vasant Lad, M.A.Sc., B.A.M.S., *is the director of the Ayurvedic Institute in Albuquerque, New Mexico.*

HARNESS HAY FEVER WITH HOMEOPATHIC REMEDIES

Homeopathic remedies can relieve the symptoms of an acute allergic attack with remarkable speed.

Homeopathic medicine comes in the form of tiny pills that are made up of extremely diluted natural substances. The substances may come from plants, minerals, or animals. With this natural allergy medicine, there's a good chance you'll get safe, effective, and rapid relief.

Homeopathy has shown positive results for the treatment of allergies in numerous clinical research studies. "But it's not magic. Success depends on exactly matching your symptoms to the right remedy," says Judyth Reichenberg-Ullman, N.D.

Dr. Reichenberg-Ullman offers these pointers for finding

the right homeopathic medicine for your acute allergy symptoms.

- The most common medicine for hay fever with watery eyes, irritating watery nasal discharge, and sneezing is Allium cepa.
- If itching of the nose and palate is your primary symptom, use Arundo or Wyethia.
- When eye symptoms (watering in particular) are your most significant symptoms, use Euphrasia—especially when your eye discharge is irritating but your nasal discharge is not.
- When your discharge is like egg white and you have cold sores, canker sores, or a headache, or you have recently experienced a disappointment, a rejection, or grief, Natrum muriaticum is recommended.
- If sneezing is your most prominent symptom, try Sabadilla.

The instructions are the same for all of these remedies. Put three pellets of the 30C strength under your tongue every 4 hours until you see improvement, advises Dr. Reichenberg-Ullman. If there is no improvement after three doses, reevaluate your symptoms. If your symptoms have changed slightly, you may need another homeopathic remedy.

For chronic allergy symptoms, consult an experienced homeopath, she adds.

—Judyth Reichenberg-Ullman, N.D., *is a naturopathic doctor, cofounder of the Northwest Center for Homeopathic Medicine in Edmonds, Washington, and coauthor of numerous books on homeopathy including* Homeopathic Self-Care: The Quick and Easy Guide for the Whole Family.

MAKE YOUR OWN SINUS-AID SALTS

A homemade nasal inhalant containing the essential oil of eucalyptus is a convenient way to clear a stuffy nose and lung congestion.

Herbalists say that the key to eucalyptus's healing power is a chemical called cineole, or eucalyptol. Evidence shows that it may relieve bronchial or nasal congestion, ease sore throats and coughs, and fight infection.

"You will find this remedy to be very handy," says herbal expert Kathi Keville. "It fits in your pocket or purse, and you can leave one in your glove box."

To make your own nasal inhaler, all you need is ¼ teaspoon coarse salt and 5 drops of eucalyptus essential oil.

Place the salt in a small glass vial and add the eucalyptus essential oil. Seal the vial tightly until you're ready to use the inhalant.

The salt will absorb the oil, but the aroma is emitted as soon as you remove the cap. Open the vial and inhale deeply. (Be careful, though. You don't want to inhale so deeply that you pull the salt into your nose.)

If the smell of eucalyptus is disagreeable, you can use peppermint or lavender instead. They're also effective.

Don't use peppermint or eucalyptus essential oils, however, at the same time as homeopathic remedies and don't use eucalyptus essential oil for more than 2 weeks without the guidance of a qualified practitioner.

—Kathi Keville *is the director of the American Herb Association, a professional member of the American Herbalists Guild, and author of* Herbs for Health and Healing.

TUNE UP WITH TUNES

You've heard the advice to whistle while you work. Music researchers say that humming throughout the day is a good idea, too, especially if your stress level is high. In fact, a hum or two could make you less susceptible to allergies.

Humming allows you to breathe more deeply and may help relieve some of the intense stress that allergies can create (or the stress that may have triggered an allergy attack). For optimal effectiveness, combine the humming with a rhythmic breathing technique.

Try this routine, offered by music researcher Don Campbell.

While you're sitting comfortably in a chair, close your eyes and gently release all the air in your lungs. Try to let out any knots or tension from your body.

Now, inhale, using your diaphragm. With the inhalation, let your stomach balloon out as you slowly count to three. Then exhale as you slowly count to six. As you do so, add humming. The "mmmm" sound can be at any pitch that feels comfortable for you. Repeat the inhalations and exhalations for a few minutes.

The exercise should be repeated as often as possible throughout the day. Campbell suggests doing it 10 times a day. At a minimum, try it when you wake up, while preparing breakfast, in the car, at work, in the shower, and before bed. These are just a few of the opportunities to practice your healing hum.

Using this technique, you relax your whole body. As you do that, you'll feel calmly alert. This exercise also promotes deeper breathing. As a result, more oxygen is allowed to enter your tissues and boost your immune system, Campbell says. Not only can it relieve breathing-related symptoms on the spot but also, when done on a daily basis, it can help lessen any future allergy attacks that are stress-related.

> **—Don Campbell** *is the founder of the Institute for Music, Health, and Education in Boulder and the author of numerous books and instructional tapes on sound and health, including* The Mozart Effect.

RELY ON AN ALL-HERBAL HELPER

With the gentle and efficient aid of herbs, you can alleviate many allergy woes.

Herbal expert Phoebe Reeve offers this impressive lineup of botanical solutions.

- The herb eyebright aids in the relief of itchy or runny eyes and drippy nose.
- Goldenrod helps to dry up mucous membranes and assists in fighting infection in the airways. (Do not use it if you have a chronic kidney disorder.)
- Hyssop helps to stop coughing spasms and can relax your nerves. As diaphoretic herbs, both hyssop and yarrow assist the body in sweating off toxins from a cold or allergy.
- Yarrow also dries up excess mucus, helps to fight infection, and soothes your air passages.

• Goldenseal stimulates the immune system. It is a deep healer helpful in cases of chronic sinus infection. (Do not use it if you have high blood pressure.)

Reeve's Classic Allergy Formula

 1 part hyssop tincture
 1 part eyebright tincture
 1 part yarrow tincture
 1 part goldenrod tincture
 ½ part goldenseal tincture (only if there is chronic infection)

Mix the hyssop, eyebright, yarrow, goldenrod, and goldenseal (if using). Swallow ½ teaspoon of the mixture in juice or water four times per day.

If you know when your seasonal allergies start, begin taking the mixture twice a day for a couple of weeks before the allergy season kicks in. Then take it as needed for as long as necessary. After 1 month, eliminate the goldenseal from the formula. After each 4-week period of taking goldenseal, you must take 1 week off.

—**Phoebe Reeve** *is a professional member of the American Herbalists Guild in Winchester, Virginia, specializing in indigenous medicinal plants and herbal education.*

GET TO THE HEART
OF YOUR SYMPTOMS
WITH FLOWER ESSENCES

An emotional issue may be the basis for your chronic allergy symptoms. If so, flower essences have the power to heal you from the inside out.

Flower essences are used to treat the person, not the disease; the cause, not the effect," says Charis Lindrooth, D.C. "Physical symptoms may come about because we store emotions in the body, so in order to effectively heal a physical illness or condition, we need to release the emotion from the body." Flower essences are one of the most effective means of facilitating that kind of healing, she claims.

Like the homeopathic remedies, flower essences are extreme dilutions of natural ingredients. "They are safe, gentle, and very effective. Don't underestimate their potential just because you take them in minute doses," says Dr. Lindrooth.

There are thousands of remedies, so write for a catalog that offers diagnostic tests or substantial descriptions of each remedy, suggests Dr. Lindrooth. The Flower Essence Pharmacy is an excellent resource. You can reach it by writing to P.O. Box 1147, Sandy, OR 97055; or online at www.floweressences.com. You can also find guidebooks to flower essences in health food stores, according to Dr. Lindrooth.

Although every person will need to carefully evaluate

himself, consider the most common flower essences for allergy treatment first, says Dr. Lindrooth.

Here are some of her recommendations.

• Goldenrod flower essence will decrease autumn seasonal allergies and will help to resolve general emotional issues associated with allergies. Goldenrod can be effectively combined with elm flower if you have a sense of being physically or mentally overwhelmed.

• Use olive flower essence for emotional or physical depletion.

• If you have a history of grief, use sweet chestnut.

• If you are emotionally fragile or sensitive to something in the environment, use lavender flower essence.

• Celery flower essence is excellent for strengthening the immune system, which is often compromised by allergies.

• Larch flower essence works well if you lack self-confidence and prefer not to call attention to yourself.

If you know you have allergies to particular plants or grasses, you may want to try them in flower essence form. These remedies may lessen, or even cure, your allergic reactions to those particular plants or grasses by helping to build natural immunity, says Dr. Lindrooth.

Once you've selected your remedy or combination of remedies, take 1 drop of each three times a day either directly on your tongue or diluted in spring water. Take the remedy 1 month prior to and during your allergy season.

—Charis Lindrooth, D.C., *is a doctor of chiropractic in Kutztown, Pennsylvania, who uses flower essences, herbs, and homeopathy extensively in her practice.*

LOVE AND LAUGH ALLERGIES AWAY

Getting at least eight hugs and three belly laughs a day can strengthen your immune system and stave off symptoms.

It sounds too good to be true, but medical research proves that laughter and hugs can be as important to the healing process as proper nutrition and exercise.

Like massage, the pressure on the skin from hugging actually decreases levels of cortisol and other stress hormones, thus improving the functioning of the immune system. Additionally, the act of touching the skin causes the body to secrete a hormone that appears to boost immunity, according to the Touch Research Institute at the University of Miami School of Medicine.

Laughter has been found to have similar effects. One study, for example, found that people who watched a 60-minute comedy video boosted their production of white blood cells by 39 percent and decreased their stress hormone levels by almost 50 percent.

"Hugs and laughter are integral to healthy living," says Effie Poy Yew Chow, R.N., Dipl.Ac., Ph.D. Aside from the scientific explanations, Dr. Chow believes that the most essential element to healing is love—and that hugs and laughter are wonderful facilitators of love's power.

There is one stipulation to the eight hugs a day that Dr. Chow recommends—they must be bear hugs. "Be sure to give and get full-body hugs—not just pressing with the upper or lower parts of the body, and no patting. A bear hug is the only hug that's like receiving a therapeutic body massage and a good dose of loving-kindness," she says.

How you get three deep belly laughs a day is up to you, says Dr. Chow. Buy a pair of Groucho glasses, make funny faces in the mirror, or start swapping jokes with your friends and coworkers. There are many free Internet services that will send you a joke every day via e-mail.

—Effie Poy Yew Chow, R.N., Dipl.Ac., Ph.D., *is a Qigong Grand Master who founded the East West Academy of Healing Arts to integrate traditional Chinese medicine with Western medicine. She is a registered nurse in public health and psychiatric nursing and a certified acupuncturist in San Francisco. Dr. Chow is the coauthor of* Miracle Healing from China . . . Qigong.

RELIEF IS JUST A BREATH AWAY

Yoga masters promise that if you practice ujjayi breathing regularly, your allergies will dramatically improve, and perhaps even go away completely.

All allergies are due to lack of *prana* (breath / life force), according to yoga masters. One way to increase your prana is by deep breathing, such as through the *ujjayi* breathing technique. Ujjayi means "to stretch" or "to extend." The extension of breath into your whole body increases your vital life force by eliminating tension and purifying your entire system, according to yoga expert Linda Rado.

Yoga experts say ujjayi breathing clears stale air and impurities from the lungs and your whole body. It slows down your internal speedometer, steadies your mind, and increases your breathing capacity. Ujjayi breathing strengthens your immune system. It relaxes, refreshes, and leaves you with a profound sense of peace and well-being.

According to Rado, performing ujjayi breathing for 20 minutes a day—10 minutes in the morning and 10 minutes in the evening—is all that is necessary.

Rado offers the following steps for the practice of ujjayi breathing.

- Notice your natural breathing pattern. When you inhale, get a sense of expansion; when you exhale, feel yourself softening.
- Find out how your breath moves through your throat. Narrow your throat passageway gently, so that you can hear the sound of your breath. Listen to the sound your breath makes.
- Slow down your breath on both the inhalation and the exhalation.
- Lengthen your breaths, so that they are fuller and slower.
- Direct the breath into your belly, filling it like a balloon. Fill the sides, back, and base of your belly and across the base of your pelvis. Continue filling upward to your waist and heart, including the ribs, chest, back, shoulders, neck, and base of the skull.
- Exhale long and slowly, also from the bottom to the top, emptying your lungs completely before inhaling again.
- Continue inhaling and exhaling, long and slowly, in a continuous flow for 10 to 12 minutes. Continue listening to the sound of your breath. Use intention rather than effort to improve the flow of your breath.

—Linda Rado, R.Y.T., *is a professional yoga teacher, yoga therapist, and co-owner of The Studio, a yoga center in West Reading, Pennsylvania. Certified in three schools of yoga, she continues advanced studies at Master Yoga Academy in La Jolla, California.*

IMAGINE BEING ALLERGY-FREE FOREVER

Allergy sufferers can bring on symptoms just by thinking about them. The good news is that the majority of them can also eliminate their symptoms through the power of the mind.

When William Mundy, M.D., and other researchers taught mind-control techniques to people with allergies, they recorded an 85 percent success rate in actually curing allergies. "Based on my studies and the positive results of research at a variety of universities, it's safe to say that imagery is a proven method for treating allergies," Dr. Mundy says.

"By combining methods called anchoring and imagery, we have a technique available for patients to help cure themselves quickly and with a significant percentage of success," says Dr. Mundy.

Imagery, otherwise known as creative visualization, is like consciously dreaming. It's created by your imagination, and it is profoundly effective, he says. Anchoring is a recall cue elicited by any of your five senses. For instance, a few notes of music make you recall an entire romantic episode, or the sight of three pine trees can anchor you quickly to a weekend in the mountains. Therapeutic anchoring is designed to deliberately associate a set of stimuli to a particular experience. Although anchoring is not necessary, it should enhance the curative effect of creative visualization.

"This visualization method will often relieve the immediate symptoms of a person having an allergy attack. It may also prevent any future suffering from allergies," says Dr.

Mundy. To visualize your relief, Mundy offers the following direction.

Close your left fist (if you're left-handed, close your right fist) and imagine yourself having an allergic reaction. Recall all body sensations you experience during an attack, such as tightness in your chest or sneezing. When you are fully engaged in the experience, still keeping your fist closed, stop the allergy image.

Now close the opposite fist, as you imagine a place and time where you feel healthy in every way. If your allergy is pollen-related, for example, you might see yourself on a seashore or on top of a snow-covered mountain. Smell the salty air and feel the cool breezes. When you see and feel yourself comfortable in every way, release both fists at the same time.

Repeat this a few times. "It seems that the immune cells, like all of us in conscious awareness, need some ritualistic repetition to make learning permanent," explains Dr. Mundy.

If you are not entirely successful, imagine a different scene where you are allergy-free.

—William Mundy, M.D., *is a clinical professor of medicine at the University of Missouri—Kansas City School of Medicine and author of numerous studies on imagery.*

Lifestyle Matters

"Once you know you have allergies, one of the easiest ways to prevent symptoms is by making small changes to your existing habits."

—Patricia McNally, M.D.,
allergist with the Kaiser Permanente Allergy Clinic in Springfield, Virginia

FLOOD OUT MUCUS

*When you're fending off allergens, you
need more water than ever.*

You may already have discovered that a 15-minute hot
shower or a humidifier in your living room can make a
big difference in relieving allergies. For the same reason, so
can drinking a lot of water.

"Water helps to thin out your mucus, which can help to
relieve congestion and sinus problems," says Wellington S.
Tichenor, M.D. By keeping your mucus thin and flowing,
you'll also help to flush allergens from your nasal passage-
ways.

Frequent allergy sufferers should drink as much water
as possible, as often as possible. Make it a goal to try to sur-
pass the minimum daily requirement of eight 8-ounce
glasses a day.

Just remember, there's no substitute for water. Fruit
juices, sodas, sports drinks, and coffee don't have the same
hydrating effect on the body as plain water.

To ensure that you're getting enough water every day,
take a pitcher to work with you and fill it up each morning.
Then, each time you drink something that isn't water, be
sure to drink one glass of water as well; or make it your goal
to empty the pitcher once a day. At home, keep a pitcher of
water in your refrigerator and do the same thing.

—Wellington S. Tichenor, M.D., *is an allergist in New
York City.*

LOSE THE MUSTACHE

A hairy upper lip is a tricky hiding place for unwanted allergens.

A mustache acts like a reservoir, providing a place for allergens to gather. And the more allergens accumulate, the more likely you are to breathe them in.

"Men who suffer from pollen allergies and who sport a mustache are at a much higher risk for developing symptoms than men without mustaches," according to Patricia McNally, M.D. She researched the effects on men who were asked to wash their mustaches in the morning and before bed. "As a result, the men reported using fewer decongestants and antihistamines, along with an increased ease in breathing, especially while sleeping," reports Dr. McNally.

Having a hairless upper lip is best, but if you can't bear to shave off your whiskers, she recommends washing facial hair at least twice a day, using a liquid soap or shampoo to get rid of pollen grains.

—Patricia McNally, M.D., *is an allergist with the Kaiser Permanente Allergy Clinic in Springfield, Virginia.*

HIT THE HAY TO FEND OFF HAY FEVER

A few extra hours under the covers may be all you need to stifle those sniffles.

As a whole, Americans are incredibly sleep deprived. Not getting enough sleep can make you more susceptible to allergens, or it can make the effect allergens have on your body even worse than they usually are.

"Sleep is the repair shop for the immune system," says Terry Phillips, Ph.D., D.Sc. "If you suffer from allergies, your body needs the time when you're sleeping to recover from the stress of the allergens you've encountered and to prepare for the stress from your next encounter with them."

In fact, in a study of people who missed 3 or more hours of sleep in a single night, the sleep-deprived group experienced a 30 percent drop in immune system activity.

"The average person needs 6 to 8 hours of sleep," says Dr. Phillips. "Anything less than that is equivalent to depriving your body and setting you up for more severe allergic reactions, an increased number of allergy attacks, or both."

To improve your existing sleep habits, Dr. Phillips suggests moving all distractions, such as a television or work, out of your bedroom. "Use your bed only for naps and for sleeping at night," she says.

—Terry Phillips, Ph.D., D.Sc., *is a professor of medicine and director of the immunogenetics and immunochemistry laboratories at George Washington University Medical Center in Washington, D.C.*

WORK OUT TO WORK UP IMMUNITY

Those trips to the gym don't just build muscle—they also build immunity.

Maintaining a strong, healthy immune system is one of the best ways to help your body fend off allergies. And the best way to keep your immune system fit, according to David C. Nieman, D.Sc., is through a regular exercise program.

"Brisk periods of exercise from activities like running, bicycling, and swimming cause an increase in the recirculation of immune cells in the body," says Dr. Nieman. This increased mobility of immune cells makes it easier for your body to fight off potential pathogens, making you stronger, healthier, and possibly more resistant to allergies.

But don't think that going out and running a marathon tomorrow will make your allergies go away. "The secret to boosting immunity is the intensity with which you exercise," says Dr. Nieman. Moderate exercise which lasts for less than an hour and a half is always best for your immune system, he says.

On the other hand, intense exercise lasting more than 90 minutes can cause your body to release stress hormones that actually suppress your immune system for several hours. That can make you more susceptible to illness—and if you're fighting a cold, allergies are harder to fend off.

—**David C. Nieman, D.Sc.,** *is a researcher in the department of health, exercise, and leisure science at Appalachian State University in Boone, North Carolina.*

WORK OUT AT THE RIGHT TIME AND PLACE

You could be causing more problems than you are solving if you don't take pollen and mold exposure into account when planning your workouts.

If you find that your allergies get worse when you exercise, you may need to make a change in when and where you work out.

"Normally, when a person breathes, they inhale about 6 liters of air per minute," explains David C. Nieman, D.Sc. "But when you're exercising, that amount can increase by up to 20 times, causing you to take in over 100 liters of air." If that air you're breathing in is full of allergens like mold or pollen, then your allergic symptoms could end up increasing twentyfold as well.

Consequently, Dr. Nieman says it's best for allergy sufferers to exercise indoors in a clean gym with filtered air. Using a treadmill or exercise bike provides the same benefits as outdoor exercise, without the increased exposure to allergens.

If you have access to a pool, try swimming laps as part of your workout. The warm, moist air in and around the pool helps to reduce the frequency and severity of allergic reactions, explains Dr. Nieman.

If indoor exercise isn't possible, at least try to schedule your jogging trips for late afternoon rather than early morning, since pollen levels are highest at that time of day.

—David C. Nieman, D.Sc., *is a researcher in the department of health, exercise, and leisure science at Appalachian State University in Boone, North Carolina.*

PRACTICE
PREVENTIVE EYE CARE

Clean, protected eyes are usually also allergy-free eyes.

When pollen or other allergens get into your eyes, the itchiness can be unbearable. But you can avoid the discomfort with some extra attention to your peepers.

"What typically happens when your eyes get hit with pollen," says Robert Plancey, M.D., "is that they become irritated and itchy, which causes you to form tears in an effort to rinse away the allergen." But if you're already congested because of a cold or other allergies, the tears can't drain away from your eyes. Then your eyes are really irritated.

According to Dr. Plancey, the best way to conquer the problem is to close your eyes and gently wipe your eyelids with a cloth dampened by warm or cool water. Repeat the procedure as often as necessary, especially when allergy conditions are at their worst.

As a means of keeping pollen and mold spores from reaching your eyes, Dr. Plancey suggests wearing glasses, sunglasses, or protective goggles whenever you're outdoors. Regular sunglasses are fine, but something with a wrap-around lens provides more protection from allergen-carrying elements.

—Robert Plancey, M.D., *is an assistant clinical professor of medicine at the University of Southern California School of Medicine in Los Angeles.*

LEARN TO BREATHE

Breathing techniques can help to reduce and prevent symptoms like wheezing and congestion.

Most yoga teachers and Ayurvedic doctors stress the importance of practicing daily breathing exercises. Since these techniques improve your general vitality, they can keep you strong when an allergy would normally wear you down.

The alternate nostril breathing technique is calming because it slows down your breathing. This helps to reduce or eliminate histamine release and other stress-related reactions going on within the body, says Trisha Lamb Feuerstein.

Bellows breathing, unlike alternate nostril breathing, actually increases the levels of oxygen within your body. The intention is to release any allergens in your respiratory system and break up congestion. When done on a regular basis, it also improves your lung capacity, giving you better resistance to the wheezing and labored breathing that often occurs during an allergy attack.

"You can initially get dizzy from either breathing exercise, especially bellows breathing," says Feuerstein. "So start out by doing one set of alternate nostril breaths or 30 seconds of moderate-pace bellows breaths, three or four times a day. You can work up to three sets of alternate nostril breathing or a few minutes of faster bellows breathing. Don't practice these if the dizziness persists," she cautions.

You can practice these techniques as long as your nasal passages are clear enough to inhale and exhale through them.

• **Alternate Nostril Breathing.** Begin by folding the first and second fingers of your right hand into your palm, keeping your thumb and the third and fourth fingers extended. Next, close your right nostril with your right thumb, says Feuerstein, and exhale and inhale carefully through your left nostril. Next, use your third and fourth fingers to close your left nostril. Release the right nostril, and exhale and inhale through it. Start the process again, closing your right nostril with your right thumb and exhaling and inhaling through your left nostril.

• **Bellows Breathing.** To perform this exercise, stand with your knees shoulder-width apart and put your hands on your knees. Practice slowly by gradually letting your stomach balloon out as you inhale through your nose. Then exhale through your nose, imagining your navel suddenly being drawn back in, making a huffing sound at the same time—as you would breathe after finishing a long, exhausting run. When you have mastered the expanding and contracting stomach movements, gradually increase the pace of your breaths. You will eventually inhale and exhale several times a second (always through your nose), like a bellows in action, for a period of several minutes.

—Trisha Lamb Feuerstein *is director of research at the Yoga Research and Education Center in Lower Lake, California.*

ENCOURAGE YOURSELF WELL

According to some doctors, whether
or not allergies get the better of you
depends on the way you see things.

As odd as it sounds, looking on the bright side of life may improve your allergies. After all, certain medical studies indicate that optimists have better immunity than pessimists. One way to apply a positive attitude to healing is to imagine yourself overcoming the illness.

Terry Phillips, Ph.D., D.Sc., worked with cancer patients who incorporated imagery into their treatment programs. "People who saw armies of white blood cells attacking their tumors ultimately experienced more favorable medical results than individuals who didn't visualize improvements in their health," Dr. Phillips reported.

"The same procedure could work for allergy sufferers," he says.

It doesn't matter how you do it, as long as you believe yourself in control of the allergens. For some people, that's as simple as picturing your allergies as a fire that your body is finally able to put out. You could also imagine pollen entering your lungs as a friend with whom you make peace, rather than perceiving it as an enemy. In other words, give it a friendlier face.

Attitude can't solve all your problems, but don't underestimate the effect it can have on your health.

—Terry Phillips, Ph.D., D.Sc., *is a professor of medicine and director of the immunogenetics and immunochemistry laboratories at George Washington University Medical Center in Washington, D.C.*

MAKE A BRINY HYGIENE HABIT

Some doctors consider a saltwater nasal rinse the ultimate practice for people with allergies, since it can save sinuses from unnecessary irritation.

A saltwater nasal rinse will help to reduce congestion, remove allergens from your nasal passages, and restore moisture to the mucous membranes in and around your nose. In the long run, it will help you avoid the sinus infections that often come as a result of frequent allergy attacks.

Here's how to do the routine, according to Ralph T. Golan, M.D.

Start out by mixing a half-teaspoon of salt and a pinch of baking soda into 1 cup of warm water. Stir the mixture until the salt and baking soda are dissolved.

Close off one nostril with your finger, then lower your nose into the salt water in the cup and sniff it up the other nostril. Alternatively, you can pour the water into the palm of your hand and sniff it from there.

If you don't like directly inhaling the liquid, you can drop it into your nose with a medicine dropper or squirt it into your nostril with a spray bottle, says Dr. Golan. If you get serious about the practice, he recommends purchasing a neti pot from a yoga catalog or health food store, which enables you to pour the solution directly into your nostril.

Whichever method you choose, inhale deeply as you sniff the solution. This may take some practice, but ultimately you want to suck the liquid up through your nostril and nasal cavities and into your mouth, where you can spit it out.

When you've finished rinsing your sinuses, very gently blow your nose to release any fluid that remains.

For maximum results, do the wash in the morning and in the evening, several times a week.

—Ralph T. Golan, M.D., *is a general practitioner in Seattle and author of* Optimal Wellness.

DON'T HAVE A PARTY ON YOUR SINUSES

Allergy problems are yet another reason to stop drinking alcohol and smoking cigarettes.

As if the threats of liver disease and lung cancer weren't enough, alcohol and cigarettes can also make your allergies worse.

"Smoking damages tiny hairlike projections in the nose and sinuses called cilia," says Richard Mabry, M.D. "These cilia sweep mucus out of your nose and prevent most allergens from entering your respiratory system." Without their protection it's easier for the allergens you breathe in to set off an allergic reaction within your bloodstream.

Making matters worse, smoke-damaged cilia are unable to do their job properly, making your sinuses much more likely to become clogged and infected.

Compounding your problems, research shows that smoking may also alter the kind of sinus secretions that your body produces, making you more vulnerable to viruses and particles you breathe in.

As for alcohol, it's a diuretic, which means that it takes vital moisture from your body.

"Excessive alcohol consumption can cause dehydration, which can lead to thicker mucus in your nasal cavities," says Dr. Mabry. And since heavier mucus can mean increased congestion, clogged sinuses, and a greater risk for developing sinusitis, people with allergies should be extremely conservative about drinking alcohol.

—Richard Mabry, M.D., *is a professor in the department of otorhinolaryngology at the University of Texas Southwestern Medical Center at Dallas.*

HEADS UP ON SLEEPING HABITS

Just a few changes in the way you sleep can leave you breathing easier.

One of the most important things allergy sufferers can do is to elevate the heads of their beds. When you lie flat, nasal drainage is slowed, and that can increase congestion and sinus problems.

Alexander C. Chester, M.D., recommends placing a couple of bricks or phone books under the legs at the head of your bed or under the head of the box spring. "You can also try sleeping with several pillows instead of one."

Dr. Chester also advises that you resist the temptation to linger in bed on your days off since lying horizontally still allows some mucus to form a pool in your sinuses, even if you elevate your head.

It's also key to sleep with your windows closed. "Pollen is mainly produced and released very early in the morning," he says, "before most people get up the energy to get out of bed and close the windows."

If you have children, another precaution is to get rid of bunk beds. A study conducted in Spain shows that children who sleep on the bottom bunk are more likely to develop allergies and asthma than children who sleep on the top bunk, since their respiratory systems may get overwhelmed by the added burden of allergens like dust mites falling onto them from the top bunk.

—**Alexander C. Chester, M.D.,** *is a clinical professor of medicine at the Georgetown University Medical Center in Washington, D.C.*

KEEP UP WITH YOUR ANTIHISTAMINE MEDICINE

If you're going to pop a pill during the severe stages of your allergy, make sure you do it consistently.

Antihistamines work by blocking histamine, the chemical that fires up your body's allergic response. A common mistake, according to William W. Storms, M.D., is using this medication too sporadically.

"One dose will make you feel better, but don't wait until your symptoms are really bad again before taking another dose. Otherwise," advises Dr. Storms, "you might feel like you're on a roller coaster."

It's best to treat antihistamine like preventive medicine during those periods when you expect to encounter a challenging allergy situation, he says. For example, take it regularly during a month when you know you have to be indoors with pets or when you're working in an area where there's a lot of pollen.

Of course, taking antihistamines all year long is too much. So if your symptoms are really chronic, an allergy shot is better—something for which you need to see your allergist or physician.

> **—William W. Storms, M.D.,** *is an associate clinical professor of medicine at the University of Colorado School of Medicine in Denver.*

DON'T WORRY, BE HEALTHY

The connection between allergy and mood is stronger than you might realize. Make resolving anxiety and depression part of your allergy-mastering strategy.

Your respiratory system is made up of numerous veins, arteries, and nerves, making it very sensitive to everything that goes on within your body. These sensitive internal connections have a definite relationship to the stress hormones that your body releases during times of severe anxiety.

"It's connected to the fight-or-flight response our ancestors developed thousands of years ago," says Sanford Archer, M.D. "If you're really excited about something, or you're under intense stress—say, having to run for your life from some animal—then your respiratory system kicks in and forms a natural decongestant, opening up the nose and making it easier for you to breathe."

"However," says Dr. Archer, "if you're depressed, sedentary, or isolated from other people, your respiratory system functions at a lower level, leaving you more vulnerable to severe allergic reactions."

If you take steps to overcome depression and bad moods, you might avoid the allergic symptoms that they can lead to. One strategy is to increase your social and physical activities. You can do this by getting more involved with friends and family members or joining a club or sports team where you can think about things other than your source of anxiety.

"The more active and happy you are, the better you'll end up feeling all around," says Dr. Archer.

Of course, if your bad mood is chronic—meaning it lasts for several months—and if it affects your ability to work or to think clearly, don't hesitate to talk to your family doctor or a psychiatrist about treatment options.

> **—Sanford Archer, M.D.,** *is an associate professor of otolaryngology at the University of Kentucky A.B. Chandler Medical Center in Lexington.*

EASE YOUR ALLERGIES AWAY

In addition to calming your mind, this relaxation technique should ease allergic reactions in your body.

Since your allergies tend to increase when you have physical or emotional stress, doctors say that any deep relaxation technique should help to reduce your symptoms and make you feel better.

Yoga researcher Trisha Lamb Feuerstein says one nearly foolproof method of easing stress is a deep relaxation technique that is part of what is called *yoga neidra.* Although yoga neidra translates from Sanskrit into "yoga sleep," the goal is to remain calmly aware, rather than actually falling asleep.

To start off the neidra, says Feuerstein, lie down on your back on a firm, flat surface with your arms spread about 18 inches away from your body, palms up, and your legs spread about 12 inches apart. Make sure you are dressed warmly enough, since you may feel cooler when you stop moving around. Once you're comfortable, begin to focus your attention on each part of your body.

Concentrate on relaxing your feet first, imagining that when you breathe in, your breath is going all the way down to your feet and melting them. When your feet feel relaxed, do the same for your ankles, and then your calves, moving all the way up your body until you finally reach your head. Consciously release tension in the individual parts of your face, including the forehead, jaw, outer corners of the eyes, and even your tongue.

Once you have completed the relaxation of all the areas in your head, Feuerstein suggests remaining on your back for at least another 10 minutes, enjoying your serene state.

"The whole process should take 20 to 30 minutes," she says, "and you should do it at least once a day, or more if you're feeling extra stressed."

—Trisha Lamb Feuerstein *is director of research at the Yoga Research and Education Center in Lower Lake, California.*

Alternative Options

If you are like most people with allergies, you've already discovered the limitations of modern medicine when it comes to treating your condition. The unpleasant side effects of prescription and over-the-counter allergy remedies alone are enough to send some people to an alternative healer for other options.

"In my opinion, conventional treatments for hay fever aren't very good," says Andrew Weil, M.D., clinical professor of internal medicine at the University of Arizona School of Medicine in Tucson, founder and director of the program in integrative medicine, and author of numerous holistic health books. "Desensitization shots are expensive, can hurt, and are risky. Antihistamines often clear up immediate symptoms, but because they act on the brain, they can make you drowsy and depressed," Dr. Weil continues. "Steroid drugs, which are prescribed for the most severe cases, can weaken your immune system over time—the last thing a person who is hypersensitive to his environment needs."

Alternative practitioners may help you recover from allergies by asking questions to identify weak links in your physical, mental, and spiritual well-being. You can then expect a gentle and soothing treatment program designed not only to resolve your allergy symptoms but to make you stronger, more energetic, and more emotionally balanced than ever.

Here's a guide to a variety of alternative healing approaches to help you select a healer or a practitioner who is ideal for you. We've also included names and addresses of organizations that can help you locate qualified practitioners in your area.

Aromatherapy

Similarly to falling in love, listening to your favorite music, or receiving a massage, the positive, relaxed state of mind from inhaling certain fragrances actually strengthens your body's immune system. In addition, many oils have specific medicinal qualities for resolving individual symptoms.

If stress seems to trigger your allergy symptoms, an aromatherapist may recommend putting a few drops of lavender oil into a handkerchief and sniffing it when you're feeling frazzled, or taking a rose-scented bath. He may give you a specific oil to use in a homemade facial steam as a congestion remedy or certain oils to rub on your chest to calm an asthma attack.

The essential oils your aromatherapist will choose depend as much on your particular symptoms as they do on what oils smell good to you. The theory, explains aromatherapist John Steele of Los Angeles, is that when a fragrance is appealing to you, you are using your body's inner wisdom to choose what will stimulate your own healing process.

On your first visit, expect a 20- to 30-minute interview with your aromatherapist. After asking about your medical history and specific symptoms, your aromatherapist will advise you on the best oils to help alleviate your symptoms and strengthen your immune system. Be sure to find out how to use the oils safely, how much to use, and how long to use them.

While some practitioners specialize in aromatherapy, it is also offered by alternative practitioners with licenses in many fields, including chiropractic, naturopathic medicine, psychology, and herbalism. You may prefer to choose an aromatherapist who is also a trained massage therapist in order to receive the additional health benefits of bodywork.

There is no formal licensing procedure for aromatherapists in the United States so you will need to check a practitioner's credentials by asking about her training.

For information on how to locate a practitioner, contact the National Association for Holistic Aromatherapy, P.O. Box 17622, Boulder, CO 80308.

Herbal Medicine

While you can follow general guidelines in a book and purchase herbal products on your own at health food stores, you may want a more personalized, in-depth treatment from a professional herbalist, particularly if your symptoms are chronic.

During your first visit, the practitioner will discuss your lifestyle and dietary habits, as well as your complete medical history—with very specific questions about the nature of your allergy symptoms and allergy triggers.

"The course of treatment for allergies must include nutritional, tonic, and restorative plants in conjunction with herbs that support the body's elimination functions," says Mary Bove, N.D., head of the department of botanical medicine at Bastyr University in Seattle.

You may initially take herbs that help to purge the allergen from your body and relieve immediate symptoms. But your herbalist will also continue to prescribe herbs for deeper levels of healing. "Allergies may be a sign of illness that is affecting many systems of the body at various levels," explains Dr. Bove.

As consumer interest in herbal medicine has grown in the United States, so has the ease of finding a practitioner. There are 15,000 to 20,000 health care professionals in this country who prescribe medicinal herbs. These include general herbalists, family doctors, naturopathic doctors, and doctors of Oriental medicine (O.M.D.'s).

To find a qualified practitioner in your area, contact the American Herbalists Guild, P.O. Box 70, Roosevelt, UT 84066.

Homeopathy

With allergy shots—the approach of conventional allergists—you're injected with a specific allergen in order to build up resistance to that substance. Homeopathic medicine takes a different approach. Rather than targeting a surface symptom, the homeopathic remedy is chosen to correct the underlying imbalance that is causing less-than-ideal health.

Emotional, mental, and environmental conditions are considered by homeopaths to be as essential to your diagnosis as your physical symptoms. They will ask detailed questions, such as whether your symptoms are better indoors or outdoors, what your mood was before your symptoms appeared, what foods you crave, and how much your nose is running. From there, homeopaths will choose from hundreds of remedies to find the right one for you.

More than 100 years of research show that the more a homeopathic remedy is diluted, the greater its potency. Since the remedies are extreme dilutions of natural substances from minerals, plants, or animals, homeopathy has earned the reputation of seldom having side effects.

Approximately 3,000 homeopaths practice nationwide, and 1,000 of them are medical doctors or osteopaths. The rest include naturopaths, nurse practitioners, dentists, licensed acupuncturists, and chiropractors. Check to see that your homeopath has completed in-depth training, which includes 500 or more hours in homeopathic philosophy, methodology, and clinical training. An indicator of those who trained intensively are the following initials in their title: D.Ht., N.D., D.H.A.N.P., or C.C.H.

For more information, contact the National Center for Homeopathy, 801 N. Fairfax Street, #306, Alexandria, VA 22314.

Naturopathic Medicine

Because of their extensive training in conventional medicine as well as natural healing arts, naturopathic physicians can offer you countless options for treatment and possible resolution of your allergic rhinitis.

They may stimulate your body's pressure points to relieve a sinus headache; give you light therapy to build overall immunity; suggest a depression-lifting exercise or a hydrotherapy routine (healing with water); and prescribe vitamin, herbal, and homeopathic supplements. Above all, most naturopaths consider dietary modifications at the core of resolving allergic rhinitis.

Ultimately, naturopaths say, a balanced diet gives you the advantage in standing up to the allergens that you inhale. Many traditional naturopathic and herbal teachings state that poor digestion creates a toxic state that leads to allergies and that respiratory problems in general are related to sluggish digestion.

Naturopathic physician Lisa Meserole, N.D., of Healing Arts in Seattle, considers a whole-foods, high-fiber diet the pinnacle of allergic rhinitis treatment.

"In order to help your body minimize its reaction to hay fever, it's essential to keep your bowels moving through plenty of fluids and a natural-foods diet," she explains. Fast food and processed foods like those made with highly refined white flour can impair proper bowel function. Instead, she recommends fresh produce; lean, organic fish and fowl; beans, nuts, seeds, and nut butters; and grains such as brown rice, millet, and spelt (an ancient form of wheat).

Request a directory of naturopathic physicians from

the American Association of Naturopathic Physicians (AANP) at 601 Valley Street, Suite 105, Seattle, WA 98109; or visit the American Naturopathic Association's (ANA) Web site at www.wnho.org/ana.htm for more information.

Qigong

Qigong is an ancient practice that attempts to bring about the harmonious integration of the human body, mind, and spirit with the universe. Derived from two Chinese words—*qi* (pronounced "chee"), the vital essence of life itself, and *gong*, discipline, work, or skill, qigong can be defined as "energy work," or "breath work."

Qigong masters, as expert practitioners are called, say that when your qi is balanced, you will effectively alleviate your allergy symptoms. Maintaining a balanced qi will prevent your allergies from returning.

While it has been practiced for thousands of years in Asia, qigong is also backed by over a decade of scientific research in the western world. Numerous studies have found qigong to be successful in the treatment of allergies. In fact, qigong masters say that their art is capable of healing where all else has failed—including terminal diseases.

If a master determines that you are extremely out of balance, he may conduct bodywork, where he may pass his hands over your body or apply pressure to energy points on your body. But the more typical approach is for him to design a series of qigong exercises specific to your health needs and instruct you to practice them regularly.

There are thousands of qigong exercises a master can choose from; some are performed sitting, while others are intricate dancelike combinations. Qigong masters will give you proper posture, breathing, and meditation techniques that help to balance the flow of qi, boost your immune system, and relax you.

"Giving individuals the power to determine and manage their own health and destinies is the secret of true healing. The healing process is a mutual education experience rather than the usual patient-practitioner relationship," explains San Francisco qigong grand master and founder of the East West Academy of Healing Arts, Effie Poy Yew Chow, R.N., Dipl.Ac., Ph.D.

There is presently no certification process for qigong masters in the United States, so take your time and search out recommendations.

For more information or to find a qualified qigong master in your area, contact the American Qigong Association at the Qigong Institute, East West Academy of Healing Arts, 450 Sutter Street, Suite 2104, San Francisco, CA 94108.

For more information on these and other alternative healing modalities, contact the Office of Alternative Medicine (OAM) at the National Institute of Health (NIH). Write for their "General Information Package" at OAM Clearinghouse, P.O. Box 8218, Silver Spring, MD 20907.

Index